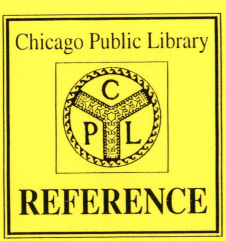

YOUR EYES

YOUR EYES

Third Edition

By

THOMAS CHALKLEY, M.D.

Shearing Eye Institute
Las Vegas, Nevada

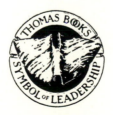

CHARLES C THOMAS • PUBLISHER
Springfield • Illinois • U.S.A.

Published and Distributed Throughout the World by

CHARLES C THOMAS • PUBLISHER
2600 South First Street
Springfield, Illinois 62794-9265

© *1995 by* CHARLES C THOMAS • PUBLISHER

ISBN 0-398-05976-4

Library of Congress Catalog Card Number: 94-45400

First Edition, 1974
Second Edition, 1982
Third Edition, 1995

Printed in the United States of America
SC-R-3

Library of Congress Cataloging-in-Publication Data

Chalkley, Thomas.
    Your eyes / by Thomas Chalkley. — 3rd ed.
      p.   cm.
    Includes index.
    ISBN 0-398-05976-4 (paper)
    1. Ophthalmology — Popular works. 2. Eye — Diseases and defects.
3. Vision. I. Title.
RE51.C43   1995
617.7 — dc20
                                       94-45400
                                          CIP

To Maggie, Dorothy and Sunni

PREFACE TO THE FIRST EDITION

In 1950 I produced a small book called *The Truth About Your Eyes*. It was designed for use by the layman interested in his own eyes, to help him understand better in a more simplified language. The book met with considerable success, and was reproduced here and in England for four editions.

The 1959 editions were surrendered to the Hadley School for the Blind, Winnetka, Illinois. In this institution the use of the book was not only for the layman, but, more importantly, it was adopted as a manual for home teachers and blind students. It has been kept in daily use since then.

The royalties rising from the sale of the second edition were given to the Hadley School in grateful appreciation of the splendid work it is doing in affording an education to many thousands of sightless people throughout this country and the rest of the world. This education is free.

The text of my book is now old. New ideas and plans are now in force. At my suggestion, Thomas Chalkley, M.D., one of my old associates, has brought out a brand new book that covers these ideas very well. It should replace *The Truth About Your Eyes* at once, and fill a need for use by students, teachers, and interested people.

DERRICK VAIL, M.D.

INTRODUCTION

The purpose of this little volume is to fulfill the need for a simple, straightforward, uncomplicated book concerning your eyes.

Vision is unquestionably one of our most important senses. We have only two eyes and they must last us a lifetime. Considering that the eye is only about an inch in diameter, it is one of the optical and electrical engineering marvels of the universe.

However, because vision is so precious, a fear of blindness is a universal human condition. If it is based on ignorance or misconception, this apprehension is unnecessary. I hope this book will help to increase the reader's understanding of the structure, function and diseases of the eye.

Fear resulting from a real eye disease is realistic. It is easier to cope with these fears and with the problem itself if it is understood. Fortunately, in ophthalmology the understanding of the difficulty can frequently lead to the solution of the problem and continuing vision and frequently vision lost can be restored. Ongoing dynamic new advances are continuing in the battle against blindness. Understanding is a large part of the battle. That's what this book is all about.

THOMAS CHALKLEY, M.D.

CONTENTS

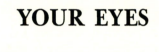

YOUR EYES

Chapter 1

THE HUMAN EYE

THE human eye is built very much like a camera, actually, a TV camera. It is hooked up to the brain by a sort of coaxial cable, the optic nerve. The image received by the eye is relayed to the brain by an electronic impulse sent down the *optic nerve.* Several relay cables in the brain then transfer the image through the brain to the *occipital lobes* at the back in which the picture is formed.

Three basic coats comprise the wall of the eye. The outer coat, the *sclera,* is of tough, firm fibrous connective tissue which gives durability and resistance to the wall of the eye. Just inside the sclera is a delicate vascular coat, the *choroid,* composed of many tiny blood vessels. The choroid's function is to nourish the inner, photosensitive coat of the eye, the *retina.* After an image is focused on the retina, which is very much like the film in a camera, it transforms the light impulses coming to it from the outside world into an electrical impulse which is transmitted by the optic nerve to the *optic pathways* of the brain.

The center of the eye is filled with a clear, jellylike substance known as the *vitreous humor.* The front portion of the eye is covered with a perfectly clear watchglass structure, the *cornea.* The cornea serves as the window of the eye.

Just behind the cornea is a compartment, known as the *anterior chamber,* which is filled with a clear fluid, the *aqueous humor.* The *iris,* which gives the eye its color, forms the back portion of the anterior chamber. Basically, the iris serves as the diaphragm of the ocular *camera.*

The hole in the center of the iris is the *pupil.* Under bright light, the pupil becomes small so that less light is admitted. In the dark, the pupil dilates widely, allowing all possible light to reach the inside of the eye. Just behind the pupil is the *lens* of the eye. It is a clear tissue suspended from the rim of the eye by many little "guy wires" known as the *zonules of Zinn.*

The zonules are attached to a little bulge in the choroid layer called the *ciliary body.* The ciliary body has some muscular fibers, the *ciliary*

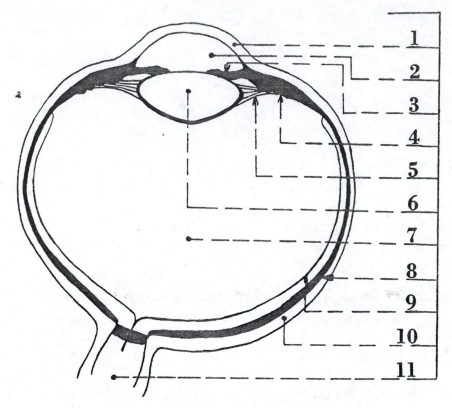

Figure 1. Simplified cross section of the human eye: 1. cornea; 2. anterior chamber; 3. iris; 4. ciliary muscle; 5. zonule fibers; 6. lens; 7. vitreous; 8. choroid; 9. retina; 10. sclera; 11. optic nerve.

muscle, which can change the tension on zonular fibers and cause the lens to become flatter or rounder. When the ciliary muscle is contracted, the lens, because it is elastic, becomes more spherical in shape. The ability to change the lens from more flat to more spherical is called the process of *accommodation.* This enables the eye to focus clearly on objects at greater or lesser distances.

The aqueous humor is secreted by the ciliary body into the posterior chamber, which is located between the iris, which makes up its front surface, and the zonules and the lens, which makes up its posterior surface. The aqueous circulates from the posterior chamber through the pupillary opening, into the anterior chamber and then flows out of the eye through the trabecular meshwork, at the angle of the anterior chamber, into the Canal of Schlemm and then on out through the aqueous veins into the veinous circulation on the surface of the eye. Except for the little

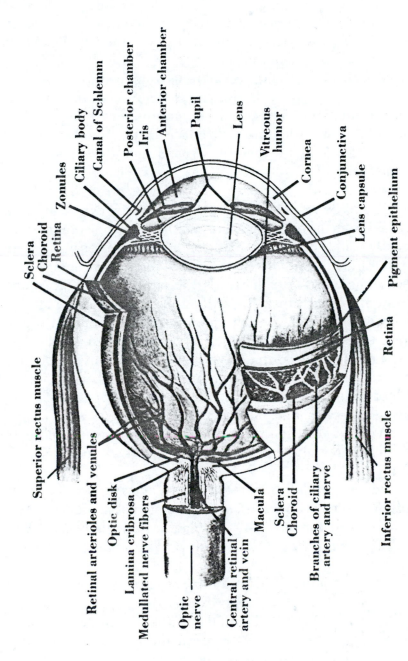

Figure 2. Internal structures of the human eye.

bulge in the front caused by the cornea, the eyeball itself is an almost perfect sphere. It is embedded in fat that is surrounded by the bony *orbit* formed by several bones of the skull. The fat cushions the eye. The hard bones of the orbit protect it from injury.

Six *extraocular muscles* move the eyeball in its compartment. They are the lateral rectus, medial rectus, superior rectus, inferior rectus, superior oblique, and inferior oblique. These extraocular muscles are responsible for the motility of the eye. All of them are attached at one end to a point on the bony orbit. The muscles' other end is attached to the sclera, the outer coat of the eye.

The optic nerve leaves the back of the eye and runs through a hole in the skull, the *optic foramen,* into the brain cavity. At the *chiasm* (Greek for X), some fibers from the optic nerve cross to the other side of the brain and some fibers continue on the same side of the brain. After making an additional connection in the *lateral geniculate body* of the brain, the fibers run back along the optic pathway to the occipital lobe of the brain.

The connections are such that the left occipital lobe receives all the visual impulses coming from the left side of each eye, and the right occipital lobe receives all the visual impulses coming from the right side of each eye. As a result, if the occipital lobe or the area just in front of the occipital lobe, on the right side of the brain, is injured, that portion of the vision routed from the right half of each eye will disappear. This is called *homonymous hemianopsia.* The right side of each eye "sees" things to the left and vice versa. If the right side of the brain is injured, left homonymous hemianopsia will result and the person will be unable to see to his left.

The upper and lower *eyelids* protect the front of the eye. They have an outer layer of skin, some deeper muscle fibers that enable them to close and open, and a deep connective-tissue plate called the *tarsus.* The many *lashes* along the margins of the eyelids provide additional protection to the eye.

Lining the inside of both eyelids is a thin, essentially clear, vascular membrane, the *conjunctiva.* It reflects back over the front surface of the sclera and continues down to blend with the *epithelium* of the cornea.

Another function of the eyelids is to push the tear film across the cornea each time one blinks. The *tears* themselves are secreted by the *lacrimal gland,* which is located just behind the outer portion of the upper eyelid. The tear film not only helps to protect the eye but it assists in keeping the cornea transparent.

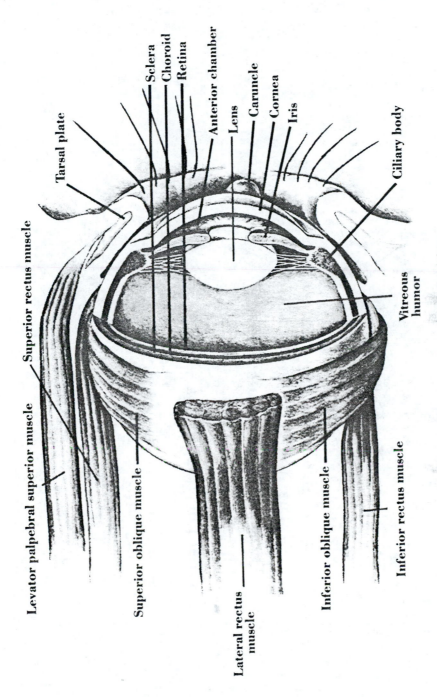

Figure 3. Side view cross section of the right eye.

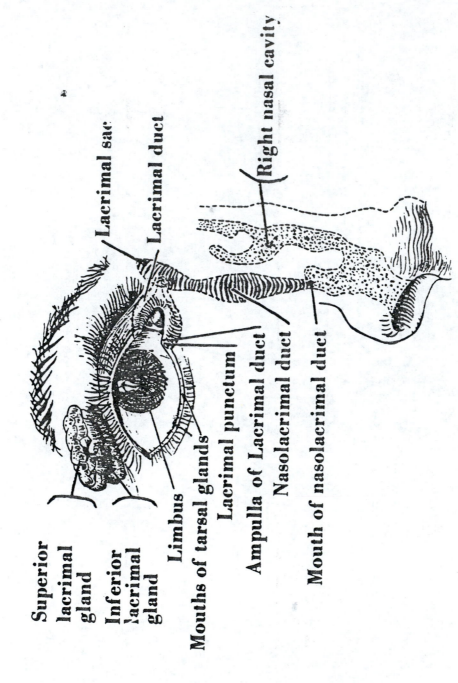

Figure 4. Lacrimal apparatus of the eye.

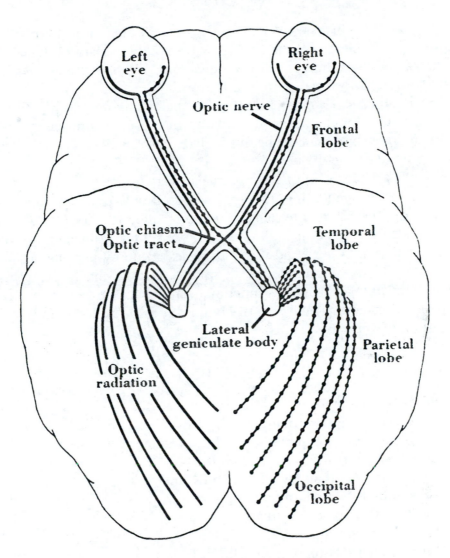

Figure 5. Optic pathways in the brain.

The tears contain an enzyme called *lysozyme,* which inhibits growth of bacteria on the surface of the eye. Irrigation of the surface of the eye by the tears and their drainage down the *lacrimal canal* to the *lacrimal sac* provides further protection from infection.

The lacrimal sac, which is located just below the medial junction of the upper and lower eyelids, drains into the nose. When one cries, or peels an onion, and the nose begins to drip, one can almost feel the tears run from the eyes to the nose.

If any part of the drainage system is overwhelmed in moments of crying or excessive tearing, the tears will spill over onto the cheeks. If the tear drainage system becomes blocked by a foreign body or disease, infection is likely to occur in the stagnant pool of tears (just as mosquitos breed in stagnant water) and it will be necessary to reopen the lacrimal apparatus. Thus the human eye, in spite of the fact that it performs a terribly intricate and complex function, is built very simply. It is merely a spherical camera attached to the brain via relay cable-obviously the invention of a creative genius!

QUESTIONS

1. What are the three coats of the wall of the eye?
2. What is the anterior chamber?
3. What substance comprises most of the volume of the eye?
4. Describe the cornea.
5. What is the pupil and what is its function?
6. What muscle is used for accommodation?
7. List the six extraocular muscles.
8. What is the chiasm?
9. What is the function of the eyelids?
10. Describe the conjunctiva.
11. What purpose do the tears serve?
12. What is the function of the occipital lobes of the brain?

Chapter 2

LIGHT AND VISION

LIGHT is energy emitted in pulses or waves from a natural (sun, moon) or an artificial (candles, electric light) source. Light travels from the sun through the vacuum of space at 186,282 miles per second. Light will also pass through a transparent object, for example, the cornea and lens of the eye. The phenomenon of vision requires that light stimulate the retinas of the eyes very much as light activates a chemical reaction in a photographic film.

The rays of light emitted from a distant source, such as the sun, travel in all directions in a formation that is essentially parallel. To provide a sharp well-defined image in the eye, these rays of light must be bent toward or focused on the retina. The curved cornea, as well as the lens, carries out this function.

Materials that permit the passage of light, such as glass or plastic, can bend the rays of light. The denser the transparent material in comparison with the surrounding air, the greater its ability to bend the rays of light because light travels more slowly through dense materials than through air. The light slows down when it hits the surface of transparent material and regains its speed after its passage into less dense air or water.

To illustrate, let us imagine a regiment of soldiers, parading across grassy ground. They reach a large, wide, sticky mud puddle at an angle. As the first rank of soldiers wade into the puddle, the oozy mud sticks to their feet. They continue marching but more slowly than the soldiers behind. As a result, the troop formation will tend to bend in toward the mud puddle. As more and more soldiers wade into the mud puddle, the entire troop slows down (a typical traffic jam). When the soldiers in the first ranks come to dry grass, they again march at normal speed away from the mud puddle through which their comrades are still struggling. Now the column of troops will tend to bend back in the original direction.

The same thing happens when rays of light traveling through air enter a piece of glass at an angle. The rays bend inward as they are slowed

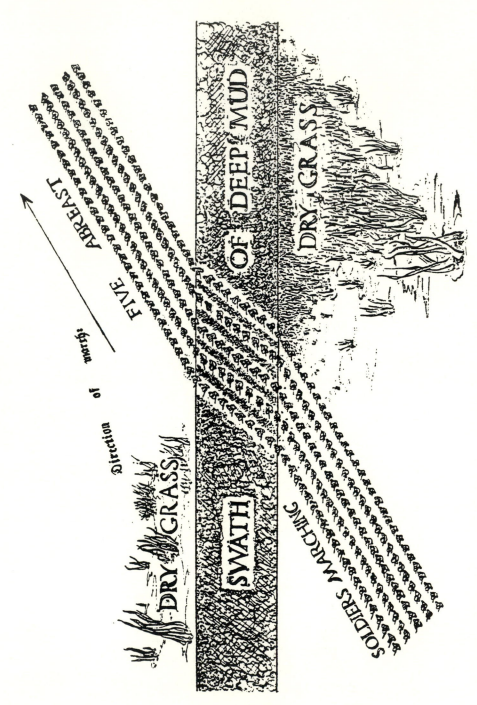

Figure 6. Illustration of analogy between column of soldiers marching through a swath of mud and the way light bends in going through glass.

down. When they exit, they bend outward. A prism of glass affords the best example of this effect. Light rays striking a triangular-shaped piece of glass, which is called a *prism,* first bend into the glass and then, as they leave the prism, bend away from its surface. The phenomenon suggests to the person who is looking at an object through a prism of glass that the image is moving toward the point of the prism.

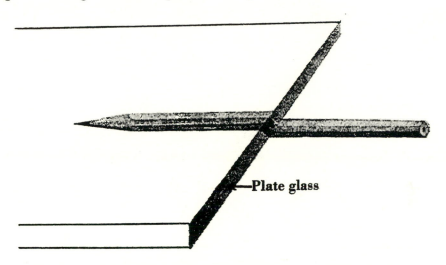

Figure 7. A pencil held behind plate glass shows refraction of light.

Putting two prisms of glass together base to base results in a simple convex, or plus, lens which, if smoothed to a more spherical shape, becomes a bi-convex spheric lens. This is merely a fancy term for a lens which is fat in the middle, thin at the rim, and rounded front and back. If the two points of the triangle of glass touch each other, the crude lens that results is called a bi-concave, or minus lens which, when smoothed until it has a more spherical surface, is called a bi-concave spheric lens. This simply means that its surface slopes inward toward the thin center and outward toward the thick rim. The effect is similar to that seen when two soup spoons are placed back to back, their bottoms touching.

Convex or plus lenses tend to bend the rays of light in on themselves and focus them at a point. The lens of the eye is of this type. Concave or minus lenses bend the rays of light away from their former axis; they do not focus the light at a point but make the observer feel that everything he sees is smaller and farther away.

If construction is imperfect and either type of lens is not completely spherical (like a soup spoon) but is warped, with more slope in the

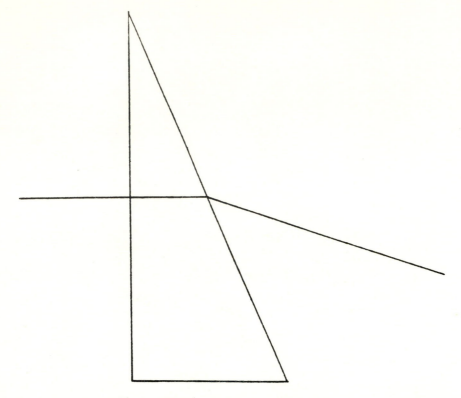

Figure 8. How a prism bends a ray of light.

horizontal direction and less slope in a perpendicular direction (like a teaspoon), the lens is astigmatic. This means that the light will not be focused on one point but on a line. The object observed through such a lens becomes distorted, just as a person strolling before the mirrors of a fun house suddenly sees an image in one mirror which is a grotesquely tall and thin caricature, and in the next is abnormally short and fat.

Placing a cylinder of glass perpendicular to the axis will correct this defect and eliminate the distorted image. The results will be a smooth spherical lens which gives clear vision.

The lens of the normal eye changes its focus automatically without conscious effort on the part of the viewer. This property is called the act of accommodation. Accommodation is the function of the ciliary muscle which is attached to the inside of the sclera just behind the rim of the iris. It surrounds the inner lining of the eye for 360 degrees. The ciliary muscle is comprised partly of choroidal material. Some retinal elements which cannot perceive light cover it. If the ciliary muscle contracts, it causes the elastic lens of the eye to relax and become spherical in shape.

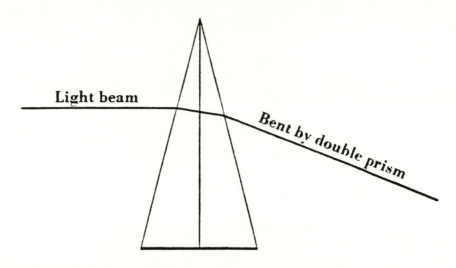

Figure 9. How two prisms back to back form the basic shape of one-half of a convex lens.

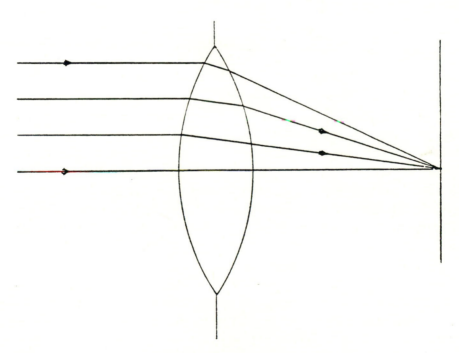

Figure 10. Prismatic power of a convex (plus) lens.

Because its surface is now more convex, it has become a stronger plus lens with the ability to focus light at a point closer to its back surface. This enables one to see objects that are closer to the eye because the rays of light emitted by near objects are no longer parallel to but are divergent from each other.

When the ciliary muscle relaxes, the suspensory fibers become taut and the lens becomes flatter, allowing a distant object to come into focus. Now the rays of light coming from the far object's surface are almost completely parallel. In the normal eye, the lens is in the position of rest. No further lens action will be needed to keep something beyond twenty feet in focus.

During aging, new lens fibers constantly develop. They compress and push more and more fibers in toward the center of the lens. This decreases the len's elasticity and, therefore, its ability to accommodate. Distant objects remain in focus but it becomes more and more difficult to focus near objects. When this happens, one needs to wear reading glasses with more convex, or plus, lens strength. This typically occurs after forty and is called presbyopia. Presbyopia generally progresses past fifty, requiring stronger and stronger glasses.

The eyes of young persons are still growing in length. When they observe close objects, light may be focused back on the retina because the rays of light are divergent and can do this. Gradually, however, it may become impossible to focus distant objects clearly, because, as the eyeball grows, the retina becomes more and more widely separated from the lens and the lens cannot flatten sufficiently to focus light on the distant retina. Such individuals need to wear concave, or minus, lenses so that the light rays reaching the eye will be divergent instead of parallel, allowing the relaxed, flattened lens to focus them on the retina.

All of this means that the person who is farsighted has the mechanism for focusing on distant objects but requires a plus lens to focus on close objects; the nearsighted individual who has an eyeball too long for his focusing apparatus requires a minus lens to observe something at a distance.

Most nearsighted (myopic) persons develop myopia in their young years while they are still growing. Their basic problem is that their eyes are too long for their focusing mechanism. On the other hand, the farsighted individual is more likely to be troubled later in life when the aging process of the lens itself no longer permits his eyes to adjust (accommodate) to close material. Farsightedness (hyperopia) affects some persons throughout their entire life, making glasses necessary even when

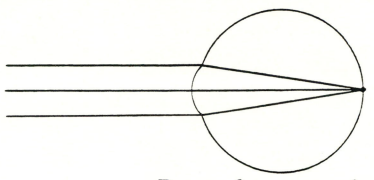

Proper focus on retina

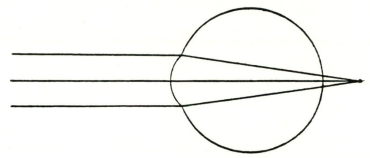

Farsightedness

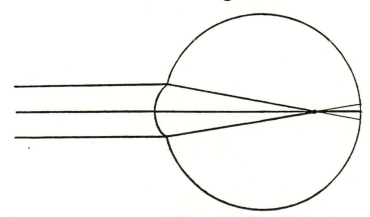

Nearsightedness

Figure 11. Optics of focus:
— Proper focus on retina (emmetropia)
— Farsightedness (hyperopia)
— Nearsightedness (myopia)

they are young. Their eyes are so short that the focusing apparatus cannot operate effectively. No matter how flat the lens becomes, light is still focused at a point beyond the retina and never on the retina itself. Only plus lenses will correct this difficulty.

When light falls on the retina, it passes easily through the inner layers on the retina, which are comprised mostly of clear nerve fibers arranged in parallel bundles, to the layer comprised of rods and cones, the photoreceptors, which lie just inside the pigmented outer layer. This pigmented layer will not permit further passage of the light.

The central portion of the retina, called the **macula,** is comprised almost completely of cone cells.

The cones are the retinal photoreceptors which perceive color. They function best in good illumination. Connected to the corresponding brain cells almost one to one by a single nerve fiber (a private line as it were), the cones are responsible for our good, clear, colorful, sharp visualization of a well-illuminated object.

The rod cells comprise most of the periphery of the retina, along with a few cones. They are connected to the brain by nerve fibers which they share with twenty, thirty, or a hundred other rods (a party line in the country). The cones are quite sensitive to light. Functioning quite well at low levels of illumination, they receive images tending to be grayish and not sharply focused. Although they provide poor color vision, rods are useful in poor illumination. In other words, the peripheral rod vision allows us to navigate in a dimly lit room without bumping into chairs and tables. The central cone (macular) vision allows us to see things clearly in full color, directly ahead. However, to work properly, cone vision requires good illumination.

Not completely understood is the way in which the rods and cones convert light impulses into nerve impulses. The most reasonable theory seems to be that conversion is due to a series of chemical reactions triggered by the light energy falling on these cells. The chemical reactions in the cones are probably different from those in the rods. Carotene, an element of vitamin A, triggers the chemical reaction in the rods. Persons deprived of vitamin A for a long time may have poor night vision, referred to as night blindness. Much less clear is the chemical reaction that occurs in the cones.

Adaptation from light to dark sometimes takes twenty to thirty minutes because bright illumination bleaches the rod vision. Adaptation from dark to light requires only a few minutes. The length of time depends on the ability of the retina to adapt to different lighting conditions as well as upon the ability of the pupil to constrict when illumination is bright and to dilate when illumination is poor.

In both situations the pupillary response is more rapid than the retinal response. The pupillary response can be extremely rapid because it is controlled by simple muscular contraction or relaxation. On the other hand, the retinal response depends upon changes in light intensities to elicit the slower chemical reactions.

There are numerous methods to test vision. The standard method, used by most ophthalmologists around the world, employs letters or figures at a distance of approximately twenty feet. Almost everyone has seen the most common test object, the **Snellen** chart, which frequently has a large letter *E* at the top.

Visual acuity is recorded in the form of a fraction. The numerator (top number) is the distance from the sitting patient's eyes to the test chart; the denominator (bottom number) is the size of the test number. Therefore, a vision of 20/20 means that the eye is perceiving at a distance of twenty feet what a normal eye can perceive at twenty feet, while 20/200 means that the eye at a distance of twenty feet is perceiving what a normal eye can perceive at a distance of two hundred feet. This, of course, is not very good vision.

Between 20/200 and 20/20 are lines of letters of diminishing size which give the visual acuity of a normal eye at one hundred, seventy, fifty, forty, thirty feet, and so on. Frequently, there are several lines smaller than the 20/20 line which demonstrate 20/15 and 20/10 vision. An occasional eye can perceive the 20/10 line. Most aviators and persons with normal vision can, under ideal circumstances, see the 20/15 line. Actually, although 20/20 vision is considered to be perfect, it may not be a normal individual's best possible vision. Often he can see better than 20/20.

Near vision is usually tested with a chart similar to the Snellen. Generally, it is the **Lebensohn** chart, which uses types of various sizes ranging from headline-size print to the considerably smaller print of the telephone directory. Type sizes are measured in points, so near-vision is recorded as ability to see four-point type, or eight point, or twenty-four point, and so on. An individual with normal eyes should be able to see four-point type fairly easily.

Since accommodation is most dynamic in young persons, eyedrops are frequently used to paralyze accommodation while their eyes are being refracted. If this were not done, their visual measurements would vary

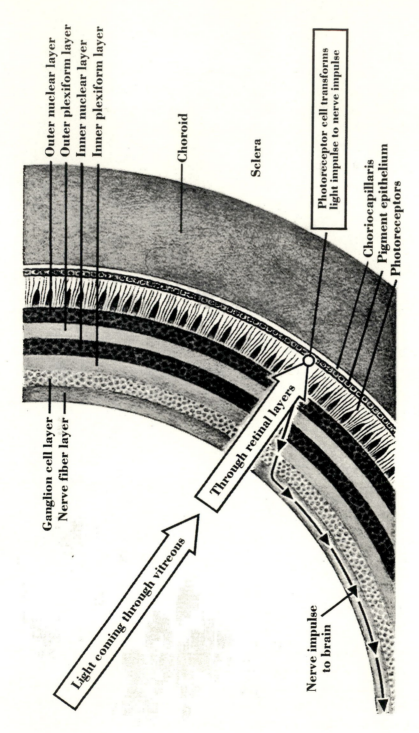

Outer nuclear layer
Outer plexiform layer
Inner nuclear layer
Inner plexiform layer

Choroid

Sclera

Photoreceptor cell transforms
light impulse to nerve impulse

Choriocapillaris
Pigment epithelium
Photoreceptors

Ganglion cell layer
Nerve fiber layer

Through retinal layers

Light coming through vitreous

Nerve impulse
to brain

Figure 12. Photoreceptors.

considerably. Unless accommodation is at rest, it is quite likely that the nearsighted patient would be overcorrected and the farsighted patient would be undercorrected.

Because the muscles of accommodation are similar in type to the muscles of the iris that produced pupillary constriction, these drops cause dilatation of the pupil as well as paralysis of accommodation.

The drugs commonly used to accomplish these two functions are atropine, scopolamine, and Cyclogyl®.

The refraction itself consists of placing either plus or minus lenses of various strengths before the eyes of the average patient until he can read the 20/20 line on the Snellen chart. However, if a patient is presbyopic and farsighted, plus lenses are placed before his eyes until he can perceive the smallest print on the near chart.

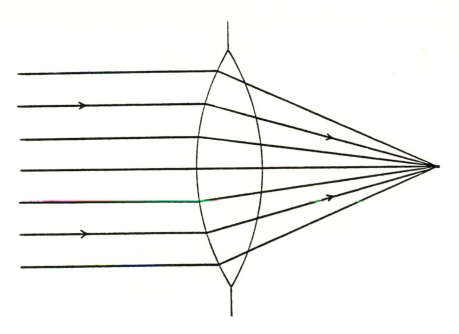

Figure 13. Refraction by a convex lens.

The refractionist then correlates the net refractive result with the patient's occupation, general health, age, and so on. This means that the glasses actually prescribed may be the same as the lenses in the trial frame at the termination of the refraction, or they may be a modification of these lenses.

It is estimated that about 30 percent of the persons who seek help for

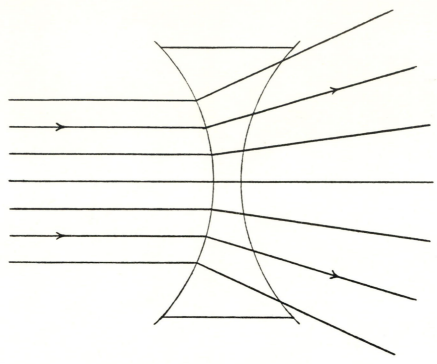

Figure 14. Refraction by a concave lens.

their eye complaints suffer some disease process which causes their ocular disorder. Seventy percent of those persons seeking the help of an ophthalmologist or optometrist suffer from simple refractive errors; glasses or contact lenses usually solve their problems.

The final prescription for glasses is written in units called *diopters*. A diopter is the strength of the lens needed to focus parallel rays of light at a distance of one meter. It requires more refractive strength to focus objects closer to the ocular lens. To focus light at half a meter requires a spectacle lens of two diopters; to focus light at one-fourth meter, a four diopter lens, and so on. All of these lenses are, of course, plus lenses.

The minus lens required to neutralize completely a plus-one sphere is a minus-one sphere; and the same ratio applies to two, three, and four-diopter minus lenses.

Correcting *astigmatic errors* requires other considerations. Since a cylinder of glass is not a perfect sphere, one must not only measure its strength in diopters, but also determine its axis.

This is very much like a silo of glass which is standing in a field. It is

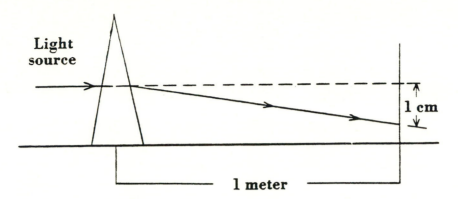

Figure 15. Prism deviation. A prism of one prism diopter strength will deviate a ray of light one centimeter in a distance of one meter.

vertical and therefore has an axis of ninety degrees. If a high wind blew the silo over to lie flat on the ground, its axis would then be one hundred eighty degrees. If it were tilted somewhere in between, as the leaning tower of Pisa, it would have an axis anywhere from zero to ninety degrees; or, if it were leaning in the opposite direction, from ninety to one hundred eighty degrees.

A typical prescription for glasses might read: plus one sphere combined with plus one cylinder axis ninety degrees; or, for a myopic patient, it might be minus two sphere minus 0.50 cylinder axis thirty-seven degrees.

After the refraction is completed, the prescription may be for glasses with lenses capable of improving either near or far vision. Older patients frequently need glasses for improving both distance and near vision. They require a stronger plus correction for reading. Bifocals may be appropriate for them.

The spectacle may be made from plastic or glass. It may be clear or tinted with one of several colors. Contact lenses are usually prescribed to improve distance vision. Contact lenses are especially suitable for patients who require a strong correction, such as very nearsighted people. Since contact lenses are worn on the surface of the eyes, they do not distort peripheral vision as do spectacle lenses, which are worn several millimeters in front of the eyes.

An older individual who wears contact lenses for distance vision must still wear reading glasses over the eye, or eyes, for close vision. Loss of accommodation makes this necessary.

At the present time, hard contact lenses are usually made of plastic. Soft contact lenses, made of silicone or of hydrophilic gelatinous types of material, are popular. Extended wear lenses, which are gas permeable (thus allowing the cornea to breathe) are rapidly gaining in popularity because they can often be left on the eye for periods of days or weeks without having to be removed.

Refractive surgery such as radial keratotomy has gained wide acceptance in the last decade. This will be discussed at greater length in Chapter 4. Also, permanent implantable contact lenses which are inserted into the eye are under development. Through a small incision the implantable contact lens (ICL) is placed behind the iris on the human's lens. It works cooperatively with the patient's eye's own lens. ICLs are intended to correct myopia, hyperopia and astigmatism in normal eyes.

QUESTIONS

1. How does light travel through a vacuum and at what speed?
2. What happens when light hits a dense, transparent surface?
3. How does a prism bend the direction of light striking it?
4. What is a plus lens?
5. What is a minus lens?
6. How does the eye change its focus?
7. What is myopia?
8. What is hyperopia and presbyopia?
9. Compare the rods to the cones.
10. What part does the pupil play in the eyes' adjustment to changes in light intensity?
11. How is visual acuity measured for distance and proximity?
12. What is astigmatism?

Chapter 3

THE CONJUNCTIVA

THE conjunctiva is a thin, transparent tissue which covers the surface of the eye, extends over the sclera, joins with the epithelium of the cornea at the limbus, and lines the inner surface of each eyelid. The bulbar conjunctiva is that portion which covers the eye itself. The palpebral conjunctiva is that portion which lines the inner surface of the eyelids.

Conjunctivitis, inflammation of the conjunctiva, is probably the most universal of all eye diseases. It is due to numerous agents, the most common of which are bacteria, viruses, parasites, allergic reactions and chemical irritations.

Since it is rich in blood vessels, the conjunctiva is quite resistant to serious damage from bacteria. Tears also protect both the conjunctiva and the cornea from infection. Not only do tears mechanically wash away invading microorganisms and debris from the eye, they also contain an enzyme called lysozyme which acts as a mild antibacterial and bacteriostatic agent.

Bacterial conjunctivitis is frequently caused by staphylococcus, streptococcus, pneumococcus, and hemophilus bacteria. Bacterial conjunctivitis may be acute or chronic. It may have a rapid onset or it may occur gradually over a period of days. It may produce violent symptoms; on the other hand, it may smolder along with minimal irritation. The severity of the conjunctivitis is often directly related to the virulence of the bacteria involved and to the general health and natural resistance of the infected individual.

Most bacterial conjunctivitis can be effectively treated by instillation of antibiotic eyedrops; the course of the disease will be milder and the symptoms will generally lessen in two or three days.

Conjunctivitis makes the eyes red, congested, and irritated. The patient on awakening in the morning finds the eyelashes stuck together with the pus produced during the night in the warm, moist area between the eye and the eyelids.

When the eyes become grossly inflamed, the patient has "pink eye", a term originally applied to conjunctivitis caused either by hemophilus or by pneumococcus. Today pink eye may be used to denote any severe bacterial conjunctivitis. However, this is more a slang descriptive term than a medical term and it is falling into disuse.

Usually, when adequately treated, bacterial conjunctivitis runs its course and clears with no threat to the eye or to vision. Occasionally, however, corneal abscesses form and heal, leaving an opaque corneal scar. Rarely, these abscesses cause thinning of the cornea, permitting the bacteria to invade the inside of the eye. Loss of the eye is then the frequent outcome.

Gonorrheal bacterial conjunctivitis (**ophthalmia neonatorum**) in newborn infants was so destructive to vision that most states passed laws making mandatory the instillation of 1% silver nitrate or penicillin eyedrops into the conjunctival sacs of all infants immediately after birth. Either of these agents will kill gonococci that invade the babies eyes during passage through the birth canal. If silver nitrate drops stronger than 1% are instilled into the conjunctival sac, the damage to the eyes can occur. Penicillin drops may cause the baby to become allergic to penicillin later in life.

Viral conjunctivitis usually occurs in epidemics. Sometimes, it is associated with a low-grade upper respiratory condition that appears to be a common cold. Inflammation of the corneal epithelium accompanies viral conjunctivitis. If staining the corneal epithelium with fluorescein solution reveals the typical punctate pattern, the viral etiology of the conjunctivitis is certain. This is called superficial punctate keratitis (inflammation of the cornea).

Viral keratoconjunctivitis (inflammation of the cornea and conjunctiva) usually is bilateral. It may be transmitted by direct contact or by swimming in pools or in contaminated water. Its normal course lasts for two to three weeks. The eyes are extremely irritated and burn. Light causes considerable discomfort. Discharge is slight. Involvement of the cornea may impair vision slightly.

Topical corticosteroid preparations may in some instances relieve the symptoms. Antibiotics may also be given to prevent secondary bacterial infection, a common complication of viral conjunctivitis.

Trachoma affects millions of human beings. Affecting all races, it is endemic in economically poor areas where bathing facilities are primitive.

It is common in China, India, the Middle East and, especially, in Egypt. In the United States, trachoma is relatively rare.

Trachoma is bilateral. It is contracted through direct contamination and contact. The agent which causes trachoma, known as TRIC for trachoma inclusion conjunctivitis, seems to have partly bacterial and partly viral properties. It is an organism that can exist only in living cells.

Mild itching and irritation are the first symptoms of trachoma. As the process continues, vision becomes somewhat blurred and the conjunctiva begins to shrink, causing the eyelashes to turn in and scratch the cornea. A layer of new blood vessels and connective tissue, called a *pannus,* invades the cornea, almost invariably from the 12 o'clock position. Small follicles form on the palpebral conjunctival surfaces and, as time goes on, scarring becomes more and more intense. Since this scarring includes the cornea, vision slowly but progressively decreases.

Eyes with trachoma are susceptible to secondary bacterial infection which accelerates the destructive process and intensifies corneal ulceration and scarring.

Treatment of trachoma consists of oral and topical administration of sulfonamides. The organisms are also susceptible to tetracycline antibiotics. Although topical medications are of value, complete eradication of the disease depends on internal administration of antibiotics or sulfonamides for three weeks.

Fungal conjunctivitis. Occasionally, such fungi as those which cause athletes' foot, thrush, vaginitis, and jock-strap itch cause conjunctivitis. A diagnostic stain and smear is the only means of identifying the causative agent. Antifungal drugs instilled in the eye will usually cure the conjunctivitis. If the fungus invades the cornea, the resulting serious, hard-to-treat corneal ulcer may progress to perforation and loss of the eye.

Allergic conjunctivitis. Almost any air-borne agent can cause allergic conjunctivitis, whether it be pollen, cosmetics, chemicals in the air, dust, or some other substance. Allergic conjunctivitis generally involves both eyes. It is characterized by extreme itching, moderate redness, thin tearing and, if the nasal passages are also involved, nasal discharge and head congestion. Hay fever and upper respiratory infections are often accompanied by allergic conjunctivitis. The disease may be mild or quite severe. If it involves the skin of the eyelids, they become inflamed, swollen, and itchy.

Allergic conjunctivitis is often self-limiting. As soon as the patient is removed from whatever agent is causing the allergy, the conjunctivitis will clear. If, however, the conjunctivitis is caused by an agent to which the patient is constantly exposed, it will become chronic and long-lasting and continue to cause considerable discomfort.

Treatment is aimed at removing the cause of the allergic conjunctivitis, if the specific agent can be identified. Cold compresses, topical cortico-steroids, and decongestant eyedrops with or without an antihistamine give considerable symptomatic relief. The condition, although annoying, seldom threatens vision.

Keratoconjunctivitis sicca (Dry Eye Syndrome), a disease often found in patients who have arthritis, is bilateral. When the tear glands become involved with the arthritic process, fewer tears of lower quality are produced and the eyes become dry and feel scratchy. They usually become red and, often, there is considerable mucus and stringy discharge. Dryness makes the eyes more susceptible to bacterial infection. Kerato-conjunctivitis sicca is chronic, generally of low grade, and always quite annoying.

Artificial tears alleviate the symptoms. If the patient irrigates his eyes frequently and applies artificial tears, he can continue to lead a normal life, and his eyes will be comfortable.

Pinguecula is a triangular patch on the conjunctiva, which occurs near the limbus, usually at the 3 o'clock or 9 o'clock position, with the base of the triangle being at the cornea. It is yellow in color and looks like a fat deposit, but it is actually due to a degeneration of the subconjunctival tissue. It is without symptoms. When the patient first discovers the presence of pinguecula, he may think a tumor is developing. It is not, for the deposit is completely benign. Pingueculae appear in older persons, cause no symptoms or difficulties, and require no treatment.

Pterygium is a small, triangular encroachment of elastic and hyaline connective tissue onto the cornea from the bulbar conjunctiva. It is frequently bilateral. Usually it invades the cornea from the nasal side and moves slowly across the corneal surface. Pterygiums affect persons who spend most of their time out-of-doors, e.g. farmers. (One of my former professors once mentioned in class that pony express riders usually had pterygiums.) As the tissue grows out over the cornea, the eyes become irritated. Eventually, the pterygium may threaten vision.

Treatment for pterygiums is surgical excision with or without local irradiation. It is not uncommon for the growths to recur and require a second or even a third excision. Although various eyedrops have been used to treat pterygiums, medical treatment is not, as yet, satisfactory.

Subconjunctival hemorrhages occur when a small conjunctival blood vessel ruptures and blood collects between the conjunctiva and the sclera. The hemorrhage continues to spread through this concealed space until a large and frightening red blotch appears on the eye. Often the hemorrhage is spontaneous. It may be a sign of high blood pressure, or it may occur in patients whose blood is too thin because of prolonged anticoagulant therapy. The condition is seldom associated with pain or discomfort. The patient may not even realize the hemorrhage has occurred until someone remarks on the fearful appearance of his eye. Subconjunctival hemorrhage causes no damage to the eye. It will absorb in two or three weeks without treatment. However, there is an enzyme in fresh pineapple which promotes absorption of clotted blood. Eating fresh pineapple could be a pleasant way to speed up the healing process.

QUESTIONS

1. What is conjunctivitis?
2. What are some of the most common causes of conjunctivitis?
3. What is ophthalmia neonatorum?
4. What is meant by keratoconjunctivitis?
5. What is Dry Eye Syndrome?
6. What causes trachoma?
7. Where is trachoma most common?
8. Can trachoma be treated?
9. Describe typical allergic conjunctivitis.
10. What is a pinguecula?
11. What is a pterygium?
12. Is a subconjunctival hemorrhage serious?

Chapter 4

THE CORNEA

THE cornea, the window of the eye, is a unique tissue. It is completely clear and avascular. A tear film covers its outside surface. The aqueous humor inside the eye bathes its inner surface. The cornea is approximately one-half inch in diameter and a little less than one millimeter thick. It is made up of five layers: *epithelium* is the outer layer; *endothelium* the inner layer. These layers are thin cellular membranes. *Bowman's membrane,* a very thin, glasslike tissue, is just beneath the epithelium. *Descemet's membrane,* similar in structure to Bowman's membrane, lies just outside the endothelium.

The main body of the cornea, the *stroma,* lies between Bowman's and Descemet's membranes. It consists of many connective tissue cells arranged in a regular pattern.

Because it is avascular, the cornea remains clear. However, lack of blood vessels makes the nutrition of the cornea unique. Most of the nutrients supplying the cells of the cornea come from the aqueous or from the blood vessels surrounding the area where the cornea joins the sclera. Additional nutrition comes from the oxygen of the air and from the tears.

Since it is an exposed structure, the cornea is susceptible to infection and injury. Any disease process affecting the cornea may make it opaque. When the cornea is injured or diseased, blood vessels may invade it. Formation of blood vessels in the cornea also can cause it to become opaque.

Dystrophies and degeneration may also destroy corneal transparency. Some of these diseases are hereditary and affect families. Any condition that reduces or destroys corneal transparency, or one that forms a scar or causes haziness, decreases vision.

Under certain circumstances, the cornea absorbs water and becomes hazy (corneal edema). This happens during an attack of glaucoma. The increased intraocular pressure forces water into the cornea. The condition can be improved by medications to reduce the intraocular pressure.

Corneal edema can also result from damage to the endothelial cells, which act like water pumps, and to some extent, damage to the epithelial cells.

Some superficial injuries to the cornea cause temporary haziness and loss of vision. However, as soon as the epithelium regenerates, vision returns to normal. When the disease process invades or involves the stroma of the cornea, loss of vision becomes permanent. No medicines will restore corneal transparency when the stroma becomes scarred and the stromal cells loose their regular pattern.

If the loss of vision is serious, a ***corneal transplant operation (keratoplasty)*** restores some or all sight. Keratoplasty is the oldest and still the most successful transplant operation. It is successful because allergic reactions to the transplant are minimal for the reason that there are no blood vessels in the donor cornea and, hopefully, no or very few blood vessels in the recipient cornea. Antibodies and antigens coming together through the blood vessels precipitate allergic reactions and cause the recipient cornea to reject the graft, which then becomes cloudy. Graft rejection is the problem that confronts surgeons who do kidney or heart or other transplants.

Present-day, long-term statistics show that an expert corneal surgeon has an excellent success rate in keratoplasties, depending, of course, on the severity of the condition causing the original corneal scar, and on the age, the general health, and the socioeconomic status of the patient.

What does corneal transplantation involve? First, the surgeon must obtain an eye from a patient who has just died. The eye must be healthy and its cornea in good condition. When fresh donor material is used, corneal transplantation must be performed within the first forty-eight hours after the donor's death, preferably within the first twenty-four hours. This gives the operation the aspects of an emergency. However, more and more transplant surgeons are using new corneal preservation materials and techniques, which enable the donor cornea to be preserved up to several days, with results comparable to those achieved with fresh material.

Keratoplasty may be performed under general anesthesia, or local anesthesia.

After the recipient has been anesthetized and his face and eye have been thoroughly cleansed, a cork bore-like trephine, ranging in diameter from six to nine millimeters, is used to remove a through-and-through circular piece of tissue from the donor's cornea. The same instrument is then used to remove the central portion of the patient's diseased cornea. The graft is then sewed to the recipient cornea with a very fine suture.

There are two methods of suturing the graft in place. Either the needle takes many small bites that are continuous around the entire three hundred and sixty degrees of the graft, or numerous small single sutures are inserted to secure the graft in the recipient cornea. Either method attaches a small, clear, round piece of cornea to the recipient's cornea.

A corticosteroid preparation is given to the patient, either in the operating room or on the days following surgery. This reduces the possibility of the graft being rejected. Local instillation of corticosteroid and antibiotic eyedrops is begun a day after surgery. Medications to maintain a low intraocular pressure may also be given. This is to circumvent the danger of water being forced into the graft. Minimizing the pressure within the eye makes it more likely that the graft will remain in position.

The patient may stay in the hospital for a few days after the keratoplasty, but more and more corneal transplants are being done on an outpatient basis and in ambulatory surgical centers.

The healing of the graft into the recipient eye is a slow process that requires several months. During this time, it is important to maintain the clarity of the graft. Any wrinkles or imperfections in the graft usually smooth out during this period. Within a month or two following corneal transplant surgery visual acuity may be quite good. The patient should not, however, become disturbed if his vision is still deficient six months after the keratoplasty. Some corneal transplants do not attain their maximum vision until a year or more after surgery.

Improvements in keratoplasty techniques, the development of newer and better suture materials and instruments and the more liberal use of corticosteroid preparations have increased the percentages of success in corneal transplantation. More keratoplasties are being performed today than ever before and this has constantly increased the need for fresh donor material. Some legislation has been passed in a few states allowing suitable eyes to be removed during autopsy, but in all cases, the next of kin should be encouraged to give permission for the removal of eyes for the purpose of corneal transplantation. Also, any adult may donate his eyes before death, by filling out a form, which is readily available at the various eye banks throughout the United States.

Some of the more common corneal affections which result in corneal scarring that requires keratoplasty are physical injuries (for example, a knife cut) and chemical injuries (lye burn). Infections of the cornea caused by the Herpes simplex virus, (dendritic keratitis) the same virus that produces cold sores on the lip, often scar the cornea. If this virus is present in the tears and causes Herpes-simplex keratitis, there is progressive degeneration of the cornea with scarring and, usually, blood vessel invasion. The cornea has no blood supply and, therefore, no antibodies to protect itself against the virus, so the same virus that causes a benign cold sore on the vascular lip can cause serious damage to the avascular cornea.

Fortunately, with the advent of antiviral medications, which can be applied topically on eyes affected with active herpes simplex keratitis, fewer eyes progress to the stages of markedly reduced vision, which require keratoplasty.

Sometimes, a serious conjunctival infection due to bacteria or fungi causes scarring of the cornea. Frequently these infections are associated with the misuse of soft and extended wear contact lenses.

Keratoconus, a condition which may cause corneal scarring, is more prevalent in younger persons, generally of teen age or in the twenties. This disease, which usually affects both eyes, causes the cornea to lose its normal, smooth, watch-glass shape and become shaped like an ice cream cone. The conical protrusion of the cornea causes considerable distortion of light. Eventually, scarring takes place. A patient with keratoconus is most appropriate for keratoplasty. The results of corneal transplantation in these cases are almost always good, and the return of vision is dramatic. Thus corneal transplantation offers a cure for the disease.

Numerous, fairly rare forms of familial corneal degeneration slowly progress until the corneas of both eyes become opaque. Generally, the victims are persons from forty to sixty years of age. Keratoplasty is frequently satisfactory in these cases. A cornea can become opaque after cataract or glaucoma surgery if the vitreous humor comes forward and adheres to the cornea, damaging the endothelium and causing the stroma to become scarred, or if the endothelium itself is damaged during the surgical procedure. Corneal transplantation frequently improves the vision of these patients.

The need for donor corneas is urgent. To fill the need, eye banks have been established in various large cities throughout the country as clearinghouses for patients who have died and whose eyes were willed for donor material. The eye bank's function is to see that the eyes from the donor are removed shortly after death, to contact the surgeon, who requests the tissue, and to transport the eye to the surgeon or to the site where the operation will be performed.

Because of the rapid improvements in corneal transplant surgery, more and more eyes which in years past would have been considered hopelessly blind can now be restored to useful function.

An entire new area of ophthalmic surgery, refractive surgery, has developed over the past decade or so. The most well-known and commonly done operation for purely refractive errors is radial keratotomy (RK). A person with myopia can be made less myopic if their cornea is flattened. This makes the cornea a less powerful plus lens. In RK the cornea is cut with a number of deep radial incisions. These incisions radiate out from the untouched center of the cornea like spokes from the hub of a cart wheel. This results in a flattening of the cornea and a number (frequently 8) of thin linear scars in the peripherial cornea. The procedure can be performed in a few minutes under topical (drops) anesthesia on an outpatient basis. The side effects are minimal and complications are unusual. After surgery the patient can frequently throw away their glasses, or contact lenses.

Corneal incisions in different patterns can also be used to reshape the cornea in the treatment of astigmatism and other refractive errors.

Similar results can be achieved by the use of lasers to reshape the cornea. This is still experimental, but may be the wave of the future.

QUESTIONS

1. Name the five layers of the cornea.
2. What is the primary purpose of the cornea?
3. How does the cornea get its nutrition?
4. Are there any blood vessels in the cornea?
5. What happens when the cornea absorbs water?
6. Is a scar of the stroma permanent?
7. What is the most successful transplant operation currently being done in medicine?
8. How soon must a fresh donor eye be used for a successful transplant operation?
9. How is the corneal transplant transferred from one eye to the other?

10. What is keratoconus?
11. What virus is the most common culprit in corneal scarring?
12. What is RK?

Chapter 5

CATARACTS

CATARACT is the term the ancients coined to describe the opacity of the human lens. They believed a cataract of water or some opaque material was spilling down inside the eye. Actually, this is a fallacy.

A cataract is not a growth of any sort. It is simply a slow, progressive clouding of the clear material of the lens of the eye, a process not unlike that taking place when, during cooking, the white of an egg gradually changes from a clear substance to an opaque, solid white one. When the lens of an eye is completely clear, it is called a *lens;* when it becomes opaque, the patient has a *cataract.* Actually both structures are the same.

The causes of cataract are numerous. The most common cause is aging. As a person becomes older, the proteins that make up the structure of the lens undergo chemical changes. Little by little, barely noticed at first, the clear proteins become cloudy, just as very low heat gradually changes an egg white from clear to opaque. It is almost certain that, if a person lives long enough, cataracts will begin to form.

Diabetes may produce cataractal changes and hasten clouding of the lens. Some cataracts are congenital; that is, "they exist in or belong to an individual from birth" (Webster). The rubella (German measles) virus incorporated into the lens of the developing embryo during maternal infection with the disease produces cataract formation even before the baby is born.

Trauma is another, not infrequent, cause of cataract. A blow to the eye or a perforating injury by a sharp object, such as a knife or pin, that penetrates the capsule of the lens changes the transparent structure to one that no longer refracts light.

Glaucoma may accelerate formation of cataracts; other eye diseases, such as uveitis or ocular tumors, may precipitate formation of lens opacities. Prolonged treatment of systemic or eye affections with large doses of corticosteroids also may cause cataractous changes.

As you may recall, the lens is a piece of avascular (without blood vessels) tissue suspended from the ciliary body by a number of minute

36

cords resembling "guy wires" that form the zonule of Zinn (a scientist for whom the familiar plant zinnia was named). The purpose of the lens is to focus light upon the retina. Like a window pane, it is useful only if it is clear. If the lens becomes clouded over, the light passing through it becomes distorted and hazy and the image projected on the retina is indistinct. As time passes and opacification intensifies, the eye with a cataractal lens can distinguish only color, light and dark, and, perhaps, the movement of shadows. The cataract is now *mature.*

Once the lens begins to cloud there is a tendency for the clouding to progress. The progression may be very slow, requiring a number of years for serious visual symptoms to occur. Or the progression may be quite rapid with serious visual loss resulting in a matter of weeks. This is more common with traumatic cataracts. The typical senile cataract tends to cloud slowly. There is no known way to prevent cataracts from occurring, or to retard their progression.

There is only one treatment for any cataract: surgical removal. No known drops, drugs, medicines, no glasses, exercises, vitamins, or magic potions will restore normal clarity to a cataractous lens.

Many cataract patients do not require cataract surgery. However, if they do, there are two basic reasons for removing the cataract: the first is to improve the patient's vision and, if no other disease is present in the eye from which the cataract is being extracted, the operation will restore useful vision in over 95 percent of the cases.

A patient may not feel the need for better vision for a number of years after his cataract has started to form. Frequently, although both eyes have cataracts, one eye may have been involved long before any cataractal changes damage the vision in the second eye. As a consequence, there are many persons with cataracts walking the streets today who are perfectly content with their vision.

However, when vision in both eyes becomes so inadequate that the patient can no longer carry on his work, get around, or take care of himself, cataract surgery is indicated.

The second reason for cataract extraction is much more urgent than the first. When a cataract in one or both eyes becomes completely opaque (termed *ripe* or *mature*), it must be removed. A mature cataract endangers the eye. It may disintegrate and cause glaucoma or iritis. It may swell and precipitate an acute attack of glaucoma. A ripe cataract must be removed before the patient is in serious trouble. Moreover, the chances of a successful outcome are greater if a cataract has not reached this stage of deterioration and disintegration which makes its extraction extremely difficult.

Exactly how is a cataract removed? The cataract can be either removed in one piece (intracapsular extraction), or in fragments (extracapsular extraction). Until the mid 1970s most cataracts were removed intracapsularly. Then several advances occurred which tipped the scale toward extracapsular extraction. One advance was phakoemulsification. A high frequency, vibrating knife is introduced into the eye through a very small incision and an irrigating port through another. The knife cuts the cataract into thousands of fragments which are washed and sucked out of the eye, this has the advantage of incisions so small that often no stitches are needed.

Another advance was the perfection of the intraocular lens (IOL) which is used to replace the lens of the eye. This is inserted into the eye behind the pupil to the same location that was occupied by the now departed cataract. The capsule of the lens of the eye has been left behind to give the IOL support. The IOL is placed in the capsular bag, which remains attached by the zonules.

The capsule is a clear membrane, like a piece of Saran Wrap®. However, it may become cloudy like a piece of wax paper months, or years after surgery. This can easily be treated by the third advance, Yag laser. The laser beam is used to make an opening in the opaque membrane. It is safe, painless, quick and effective.

The use of laser in treating the postcataract membrane has caused a misconception to be widely circulated, that laser is used to remove cataracts. Cataracts *cannot* be removed by laser surgery.

The advantages of extracapsular cataract extraction now far outweigh those of intracapsular. The surgery is simpler, quicker and safer than intracapsular. Rehabilitation is faster. As a result, almost all cataract surgery is now performed on an outpatient basis.

What does a cataract operation involve? After sedation, the patient is taken to the operating room where the eye is anesthetized. The local anesthetic deadens all sensation and eliminates the possibility of the patient feeling pain, although he is awake and capable of cooperating with the surgeon. Rarely is it necessary to administer a general anesthetic.

While the anesthetic is taking effect, the patient's face and eye are thoroughly cleaned with surgical soap, and a drape is placed. After the anesthetic has taken effect, the surgery is performed. Generally, the operation takes 15 or 20 minutes to perform. Then an antibiotic solution or ointment and, sometimes, a corticosteroid ointment are applied to the eye which is then covered with a dressing. The operation is over.

The patient is returned to a waiting area for a short period of observation. Then he returns home. The next week is spent convalescing and heavy physical activity should be avoided.

When a cataract is removed, the lens of the eye is being removed. Hence, after the eye is recovered, some optical compensation must be made for the loss of the lens. This can be done in one of three ways: with glasses, with a contact lens, or with an intraocular lens inserted into the eye, either at the time of the cataract extraction or at a later date.

When I took my residency in ophthalmology a third of a century ago, almost everyone who had cataract surgery received cataract glasses. These were thick magnifying glasses which caused lots of getting used to and most people who wore them were more or less handicapped by the peripheral distortion and the enormous magnification. As improvements were made in cataract lenses over the next decade or so, more and more people switched to contacts. However, they require a certain amount of dexterity in handling and many elderly people have a very difficult time inserting and removing contacts. And when they are removed, cataract glasses are still needed. Theoretically, the most normal place to wear a lens is actually inside the eye behind the pupil, in the exact location where the normal lens of the eye resides. Great advances have been made in the last decade in intraocular lenses. They were first used after World War II, in England, but so many problems were encountered with the original intraocular lenses that approximately two decades went by, between the late 1940s and late 1960s, when they were held in general disfavor by the ophthalmic community. However, new lenses were developed in the 1960s and 1970s, which were of more durable material, lighter in weight, and designed to be less irritating and more readily accepted by the eye, and now intraocular lens implantation has become the treatment of choice and has gained universal acceptance.

Although it is a nuisance to have to undergo cataract surgery, it is generally one of the safest and most successful of all operations, truly a miracle of modern surgery. Therefore, the person who has cataracts should not despair, but put himself in the hands of a competent ophthalmologist who will follow the progress of the cataracts and, if it becomes necessary, remove them and restore his vision.

QUESTIONS

1. What is a cataract?
2. How does a cataract differ from the lens of the eye?
3. Why does a person with cataracts have trouble seeing?
4. What is a *mature* cataract?
5. Can cataracts generally be prevented?
6. What is the treatment for cataracts?
7. Give two primary reasons for removing cataracts.
8. What is an IOL?
9. If you were to have cataract surgery would you prefer to have cataract glasses, or IOL?

Chapter 6

GLAUCOMA

GLAUCOMA is a disease in which the pressure of the eye rises to a point where it causes damage to the optic nerve. The optic nerve has small, soft, and tender fibers. As these fibers leave the back of the eye, the tough scleral covering of the eye directly surrounds the fibers. If the pressure in the eye rises so that the peripheral fibers are squeezed against the hard sclera, the fibers will die. The rise in pressure will also compromise their fragile blood supply.

Nature will then remove the dead fibers and the undamaged more centrally located nerve fibers will be forced against the tough sclera. These fibers, too, will die. Bit by bit, the peripheral vision of the eye deteriorates and disappears. Bit by bit, the field of vision becomes narrower. Finally, the only nerve fibers remaining are those in the very center of the nerve. They are the fibers that supply the center of the retina, the macular area, and provide good central vision. Because of this, central reading vision is the last portion of vision to be involved by glaucoma.

The patient suffering from glaucoma, whose intraocular pressure is not so high as to cause pain but is sufficiently high to damage the optic nerve, slowly becomes blind, unaware of the loss of his peripheral vision; only when his central vision begins to disappear and he has difficulty reading does he finally seek assistance.

The incidence of this insidious type of glaucoma, which is termed *chronic open-angle glaucoma,* is much higher than that of any other form of glaucoma. Generally, the condition involves both eyes simultaneously. The patient may not realize that he is going blind until it is too late, for both eyes may be severely damaged before he consults an ophthalmologist.

One way of diagnosing chronic open-angle glaucoma is to measure the intraocular pressure. Normal pressures range from ten to twenty-four millimeters of mercury. The eye requires a pressure to keep it round and the cornea smooth. Without pressure the eye would collapse like a leaky balloon. However, measurements higher than twenty-four millimeters of

Hg (mercury) suggest the presence of glaucoma. Readings in the thirty to forty millimeter Hg range or higher indicate definite glaucoma.

A second way to diagnose glaucoma is to do visual field studies, which will reveal typical glaucoma defects in peripheral vision. One of the early field changes is an enlargement of the normal blind spot.

Other forms of glaucoma may be just as serious or even more serious than chronic open-angle glaucoma. However, they are easier to diagnose.

The most spectacular type of glaucoma is known as *angle-closure* or *narrow-angle glaucoma.* It occurs in a person who has probably had no trouble with his eyes until he suddenly suffers severe, agonizing pain in one or both eyes. As water is forced into the cornea, vision becomes dim. Light hitting the water in the steamy cornea causes the patient to see rainbowlike halos. The eye becomes red, congested, and rock-hard. The intraocular pressure rises to sixty, seventy, eighty, or even as high as one hundred and twenty millimeters Hg.

All of these critical events can occur over the course of a few hours. Usually the patient seeks immediate help to relieve the pain and blindness. If he doesn't, he should, for time is of the essence when acute glaucoma strikes.

Congenital and *secondary glaucoma* are two forms of this destructive disease which are less spectacular but just as dangerous.

If a child is born with an improperly formed ocular drainage system, the increased intraocular pressure causes the eye to stretch because the connective tissue in the sclera and cornea are still pliable during the first few months of life. These babies have very large and beautiful eyes. Unless they are treated, however, they will become blind.

Secondary glaucoma, as the name implies, is triggered by some other ocular disease process that interferes with the drainage system of the eye. The culprit could be cataract, injury, infection, iritis, or almost any other eye affection. If the underlying eye disease is treated successfully, the glaucoma usually is cured. Glaucoma may also be secondary to the use of medications such as corticosteroids.

Causes of Glaucoma

Basically, glaucoma is a plumbing problem. The aqueous humor, as you recall, is secreted by the ciliary body. It circulates through the posterior chamber of the eye, out through the pupil, and into the anterior chamber. It then circulates through the *trabecular meshwork* and the *canal of Schlemm* before the *aqueous veins* remove it and return it to the venous circulation.

Most glaucomas reflect a resistance to outflow of aqueous through the trabecular meshwork and the canal of Schlemm at the angle of the eye. The *angle of the eye,* formed by the junction of the iris with the inside of the cornea and sclera, extends around the entire 360 degrees of the eye.

The trabecular meshwork overlies the canal of Schlemm. It is a sieve-like structure with numerous little holes. Although the trabecula allows aqueous to drain through, it is rather resistant to the drainage. In this respect, it resembles a sink drain that is covered with a permanent sieve to catch refuse. If the sink sieve becomes blocked or plugged, naturally the water level in the sink rises.

Blockage of drainage from the eye presents a more complex problem. The eye is a rigid, closed-in structure in which the water level cannot rise. Only the pressure of the water rises in an attempt to force the customary amount of fluid through the ocular drain. The increased pressure damages the optic nerve and its blood supply.

In chronic open-angle glaucoma, the mechanism of drainage stoppage is not clearly understood. It is known that stoppage occurs at the trabecular meshwork and the canal of Schlemm and that the increased resistance to aqueous drainage from the eye slowly elevates the intraocular pressure.

In acute closed-angle glaucoma, the iris is too far forward toward the cornea and virtually lies over the drainage system. Dilatation of the pupil by fright or by sitting in a darkened room, or whatever, thickens the root of the iris. Now it completely covers the drain. As the iris is forced farther and farther into the drain, the intraocular pressure rises with increasing rapidity. In the narrow-angle eye, the more firmly the iris is forced into the trabecular meshwork, the higher the intraocular pressure becomes. If untreated, the pressure within the eye will rise astronomically in a very short time, causing blindness within a few hours or a few days. The pain is extreme, and the anxiety of the patient is intense, as it should be.

In secondary glaucoma, white blood cells, red blood cells, cortical debris from a broken cataract, blood vessels in a patient with diabetes, or a swollen cataract mechanically block the drain. A tumor of the eye may swell and block the trabecular meshwork. Any of these occurrences increase the intraocular pressure. If the underlying disease is controlled or cured, usually drainage will be reestablished and the pressure will return to normal levels.

Treatment of Glaucoma

In primary open-angle glaucoma, the usual treatment is to constrict the pupils with eyedrops and prescribe medicine used to reduce water retention. *Pilocarpine* is a commonly-used topical medication for constricting the pupil so that the iris will be pulled from the trabecular meshwork and thereby increase drainage. Pilocarpine may also decrease the amount of aqueous entering the eye from the ciliary body. When the pupil is small, the iris is stretched out to its maximum surface so that it absorbs fluids more readily and removes them from the eye, thus affording a secondary drainage channel.

Other eyedrops, similar to pilocarpine in therapeutic action, may be stronger or may function through slightly different chemical mechanisms. *Epinephrine* is another antiglaucoma eyedrop. It produces some dilation of the pupil, which is not dangerous in open-angle glaucoma, and definitely decreases the amount of aqueous coming into the eye. However, it is very dangerous to use in a narrow-angle eye.

Beta adrenergic blocking agents have a similar effect on open angle glaucoma but have fewer of the topical side effects of epinephrine. However, they should be used with caution with patients who have certain cardiac or respiratory difficulties. Timolol® is a commonly prescribed beta blocker.

Diamox®, a diuretic, and similar preparations are taken internally to decrease aqueous production by the secretory cells of the ciliary body.

In an occasional case of open-angle glaucoma, it is necessary to perform a *filtering operation.* A hole is made through the sclera at the angle of the anterior chamber to create a channel for the aqueous to drain from the anterior chamber out underneath the conjunctiva. This operation may be done with or without the incorporation of a mechanical valve. This surgery is usually incorporated with some form of iridectomy. In this operation, a hole is made through the periphery of the iris. Occasionally, when filtering operations do not work satisfactorily, such methods as diathermy or cryothermy (freezing) to the ciliary body will bring about decrease of aqueous formation.

In narrow-angle glaucoma, the same medical treatment described for open-angle glaucoma (pilocarpine eyedrops and oral Diamox) is used to try to temporarily reduce the intraocular pressure. In addition, glycerine, a potent dehydrating agent, is given orally, or manitol, which has a similar effect, may be given intravenously. Glycerine produces a very rapid reduction in the intraocular pressure. However, its action is transient. As soon as the pressure in narrow-angle glaucoma has been lowered to a more normal range, a *peripheral iridectomy* is performed adjacent to the angle. The small hole that is made in the iris never heals. Because the hole always remains open, the aqueous can drain directly from the posterior chamber into the drainage area of the anterior chamber instead of having to make the longer trip through the pupil. Not only is the iris no longer pushed forward to obstruct the trabecular meshwork but also one portion of the ocular drainage system will always be exposed to the aqueous. The iris can never block the angle in the area of the iridectomy. Iridectomy usually effects a complete cure of closed-angle glaucoma. Frequently, after the operation, eyedrops will no longer be needed. In most cases of closed-angle glaucoma both eyes are involved. Because of this, if an acute attack occurs in one eye, a prophylactic peripheral iridectomy should be performed on the second eye. If the hole in the iris is made with a laser it is called *peripheral iridotomy*. Because the laser can be used in an office setting, obviating a trip to the operating room, laser iridotomies have become popular.

In congenital glaucoma, the drain has never opened properly and a persistant membrane overlies the trabecular meshwork, blocking the drainage system and keeping the aqueous from flowing out. The aim of an operation in these cases is to open the membrane so that the trabecular meshwork will become bathed in aqueous. An extremely sharp knife is thrust through the cornea into the angle of the chamber. Under direct visualization, the congenital membrane is cut. It then retracts, leaving a gaping hole. The angle is now open. If cutting the congenital membrane does not suffice, a filtering operation has to be performed.

Although, in secondary glaucoma, the basic treatment is to alleviate the condition causing the increased intraocular pressure, frequently drops and oral Diamox are needed to control the pressure while the cause is being treated.

Glaucoma Is a Frightening Disease.

Thousands of persons are unaware that they have chronic open-angle glaucoma and are gradually losing their sight. They have no pain to warn them that something is wrong with their eyes. Treatment is the only help for the glaucoma patient. The only way to avert the disaster of blindness is to have the intraocular pressure checked regularly. *Tonometry* (measuring the intraocular pressure) is a simple procedure. It requires only a few seconds and is painless. Almost all glaucoma patients can be helped, further damage to the eyes can be avoided, and blindness can be thwarted.

Everyone over the age of forty years should visit an ophthalmologist once a year to have his intraocular pressure checked.

QUESTIONS

1. What is glaucoma?
2. What structure does glaucoma damage?
3. List four types of glaucoma.
4. What type of glaucoma is the most insidious and furtive?
5. What type of glaucoma is the most explosive and why?
6. Describe the circulation of aqueous from the ciliary body to aqueous veins.
7. What is the basic mechanism of closed-angle glaucoma?
8. What medicines are used to treat open-angle glaucoma?
9. What is a filtering operation?
10. What operation is used to treat narrow-angle glaucoma?
11. What is the basic structural problem in congenital glaucoma?
12. What are some causes of secondary glaucoma?

Chapter 7

THE UVEAL TRACT

THE choroid, ciliary body, and iris make up the *uveal tract,* the middle vascular layer of the eye. Externally, the uveal tract adheres to the sclera; internally, it adheres to the retina. The *iris* is the most familiar and easily visible portion of the uveal tract.

The iris, the *colored* portion of the eye, forms the posterior border of the anterior chamber and the anterior border of the posterior chamber. It is a rather flat, flexible tissue that surrounds the *pupil,* an aperture (opening) in its center.

The size of the pupil varies as the iris dilates and constricts. When the pupil is widely dilated, very little of the iris is visible. When the pupil is constricted, almost all of the iris is visible. Dilation and constriction are accomplished by the *dilator* and *sphincter* muscles in the iris.

The amount of pigmentation present in the iris determines its color, whether gray, green, blue, or brown. The greater the pigmentation, the darker the iris and the darker the eye appears.

Two interesting characteristics of the iris are that, although it is a highly vascular structure, when cut it seldom bleeds, and any hole formed in the iris will not heal shut.

The root of the iris is attached to the *ciliary body,* a somewhat elevated structure which runs 360 degrees around the inside of the eye. The ciliary body is not readily visible to the observer, since it is located beneath the white of the eye and just behind the root of the iris. The lens is suspended from the inner surface of the ciliary body by little "guy wires" called the *zonules of Zinn.* In addition, the ciliary body has the secretory function of producing aqueous humor.

Most of the ciliary body is composed of muscle fibers which, on contracting and relaxing, change the shape of the lens, allowing the eye to focus at different points in the distance. This phenomenon is called *accommodation.*

The *choroid,* the other part of the uveal tract, lies between the retina and sclera. It is a vascular structure that supplies the outer layers of the retina with most of their nutrition.

Iritis

Inflammation of the iris is called *iritis*. As with other inflamed structures in the body, movement of the iris is accompanied by pain. One of the first signs of iritis is *photophobia* (fear of light): when bright light is shone into the eye constriction of the pupil stretches the tender and inflamed iris and produces pain. Patients suffering from iritis are extremely sensitive to bright light.

Inflammation of the iris may cause congestion beneath the sclera, observed as **ciliary flush**. A deep ring of inflammation surrounds the limbus and the area just posterior to the limbus. As the inflammation continues, the blood vessels in the iris begin to extrude white blood cells and protein into the aqueous. The normal, watery aqueous becomes thick, sticky, and syrupy. Shining a beam of light into the anterior chamber illuminates the individual white cells which, when observed with a microscope, resemble the individual snowflakes caught in the illumination from automobile headlights during a snow storm. This feature distinguishes iritis, and the ophthalmologist can confirm his diagnosis when he examines the eye with a microscope attached to a beam of light in an instrument called a **slitlamp**.

As white blood cells circulate in the anterior chamber, some become stuck to the back of the cornea. These are known as **keratitic precipitates** (or KP's).

Although the intraocular pressure decreases in some patients suffering from iritis, probably because the inflamed ciliary body produces less aqueous, in other cases of iritis, the white cells and protein clog the outflow drains at the angle of the eye and cause increased intraocular pressure and secondary glaucoma.

Iritis can also cause formation of adhesions where the pupillary edge of the iris touches the anterior capsule of the lens because the sticky proteinaceous material circulating in the anterior chamber acts like glue. Such adhesions may be permanent; strong dilation of the pupil will not break them. Early dilation of the pupil in a case of iritis usually pulls the iris far enough away from the anterior surface of the lens so that adhesion is averted.

Peripheral adhesions may also form between the anterior surface of

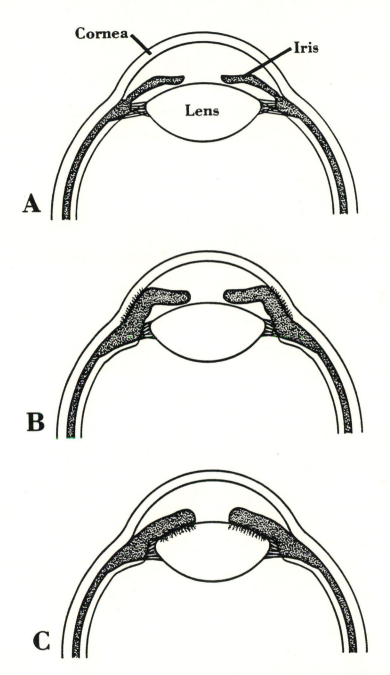

Figure 16. Uveitis. A. Normal iris-corneal angle. B. Anterior synechias (adhesions): The peripheral iris adheres to the cornea. C. Posterior synechias: the iris adheres to the lens.

the root of the iris and the posterior surface of the margin of the cornea at the angle. If there are enough peripheral adhesions to block the angle, the intraocular pressure will become markedly elevated and severe secondary glaucoma will ensue.

The exact cause of iritis is unknown. Many persons who suffer from rheumatoid arthritis and associated types of joint disease have iritis. The ocular disease may also be associated with tuberculosis, sarcoidosis, and syphilis. It may also accompany toxoplasmosis and other infectious diseases. Many cases of iritis, however, are probably not due to direct infection by bacteria or viruses but to a secondary allergic reaction to some organism or to some disease process in the body.

Occasionally, iritis occurs secondary to extrusion of lens material into the aqueous through a ruptured lens capsule. The iris becomes hypersensitive to the protein of the lens and *lens-induced* iritis is the consequence. Occasionally, too, when the uveal tract has been involved in an eye injury, the body acquires hypersensitivity to the material of the uveal tract, possibly to the uveal pigment. This reaction of the body to its own uveal pigment can cause a sudden and extremely dangerous type of uveitis in both the injured and uninjured eye. This phenomenon is called *sympathetic ophthalmia.*

Sympathetic ophthalmia will not develop if the severely injured eye is removed within ten days of the injury. In order to save the uninjured eye, it is necessary to remove the severely injured eye for which there is no hope of regaining vision. Sympathetic ophthalmia can occur at any time from two weeks to twenty-five years after the injury.

The treatment of iritis is aimed at preventing the formation of adhesions between the iris and the lens by dilating the pupil. Heat reduces the pain frequently present in iritis. Salicylates (aspirin) often benefit the patients, especially those who have rheumatoid arthritis.

Corticosteroid medication, taken topically as eyedrops and systemically, is the most valuable treatment for iritis. Corticosteroids do not cure the disease process: they simply protect the eye from the inflammatory reaction until the cause of the iritis burns itself out. This may occur in a few days or drag on for years.

Choroid

The two primary disease processes affecting the choroid are malignant melanoma and choroiditis.

Malignant melanoma of the choroid, the most common malignant intraocular tumor, generally affects Caucasians and older individuals. It is extremely rare in blacks. The average age of patients suffering from choroidal malignant melanoma is fifty years. It almost always involves one eye only. Approximately 85 percent of malignant melanomas of the eye arise in the choroid; the remaining 15 percent occur in the ciliary body and the iris.

In its early stages, a malignant melanoma may be discovered by accident during a routine ophthalmological examination. As the size of the tumor increases, vision may become blurred. Fortunately, the tumor usually does not spread from the eye until fairly late in its development.

Removal of the eye, hopefully before the tumor spreads to the liver, brain, or other structures of the body, is the treatment for malignant melanoma of the eye. If the tumor in the eye is removed in its entirety before it has spread to other structures, there is probably no threat to life. Sometimes, however, distant metastases are not discovered until a number of years after the eye has been enucleated. Occasionally radiation and chemotherapy are used in the treatment of malignant melanoma.

Approximately 50 percent of the patients who have had one eye removed for malignant melanoma survive five years. This is not an encouraging statistic; nevertheless, if it is compared with the statistics for cases of malignant melanoma elsewhere in the body (which are usually fatal), it is somewhat heartening.

Unfortunately, the eye that is removed because of a presumptive diagnosis of malignant melanoma often has relatively good vision. If the diagnosis is wrong, a reasonably good eye has been sacrificed. However, malignant melanoma is usually correctly diagnosed.

When a malignant melanoma occurs in the iris or ciliary body, it is usually discovered early and removed together with a surrounding portion of the iris and ciliary body. In these cases, it is not necessary to remove the entire eye.

Choroiditis, an inflammation of the choroid, is most commonly due to one of several infectious agents. Among the offenders are tuberculosis, syphilis, sarcoid, toxoplasmosis, and histoplasmosis. Unlike hypersensitive reactions in the iris, the agent is usually present in the choroid itself. Determination of the specific agent, however, frequently poses a dilemma. Direct biopsy of the choroid to localize and identify the causative agent is contradicted because the biopsy itself would cause severe damage to the eye. Since such a definitive diagnostic procedure is more dangerous than the disease process itself, the ophthalmologist must rely primarily on the clinical picture and blood and skin tests to make his diagnosis.

If the cause of the choroiditis appears to be tuberculosis, antitubercular drugs are administered. If sarcoidosis is diagnosed, corticosteroids are of value. If toxoplasma are implicated, other medications are effective. In the fungus infection histoplasmosis, amphotericin B may be helpful, although it is seldom used because it is very toxic. Systemic corticosteroid preparations may be of some value in the treatment of histoplasmosis and laser has been used.

When choroiditis involves the peripheral choroid, any resulting defect in the peripheral field of vision should not interfere greatly with the efficiency of the eye. On the other hand, if chorioretinitis involves the macular area, there may be extreme loss of central vision to as much as 20/200 or finger counting, considerably handicapping the efficiency of the eye.

QUESTIONS

1. What is the uveal tract?
2. What are the two muscles that move the iris?
3. What gives the iris its color?
4. What are the two basic functions of the ciliary body?
5. What is the basic function of the choroid?
6. What is iritis?
7. What is a KP?
8. How can iris adhesions cause secondary glaucoma?
9. What are some things that cause iritis?
10. What is sympathetic ophthalmia?
11. What is a malignant melanoma?
12. What is choroiditis?

Chapter 8

THE RETINA

THE retina, the internal lining of the wall of the eye, is equivalent in function to the film of a camera. It is the function of the cornea and lens to focus light on the retina and the function of the sclera and choroid to protect and nourish the retina, so that it can perceive an image and relay the picture by way of the optic nerve to the brain. In a sense, the retina, therefore, is the most vital tissue in the eye because it is the only tissue that is photosensitive.

The retina is nourished by blood vessels which come through the optic nerve and run across its inner surface. The choroid, the next outermost layer of the eye, also supplies the retina with nourishment.

The retina is an extremely delicate and sensitive tissue. If it is deprived of its blood supply for more than a few minutes, it dies and cannot be replaced.

The central portion of the retina, the macula, a small area about one-half millimeter in diameter, is used for extremely fine, sharp, colorful vision. To get the best picture of an image, one unconsciously endeavors to focus it on the macula.

Of the two basic types of photoreceptors in the retina, the *rods* and the *cones,* the cones almost exclusively occupy the macular area. A sharp, clear picture and good color vision depend on the cones which, in turn, depend on light of rather high intensity to achieve a good picture.

The peripheral retina, composed almost entirely of rods, provides excellent night vision, although the images it relays to the brain are less distinct, detailed, and colorful than those transmitted by the cones.

Inside the retina and occupying the entire center of the eye is the vitreous humor or vitreous body, a clear, jellylike material. Although the vitreous may be attached to the retina at a number of points, almost invariably it is attached to the optic nerve and to that portion of the retina just behind the ciliary body.

The ophthalmologist is able to examine the retina through an ophthalmascope, an instrument which consists of a light source and a lens,

53

through which the observer looks into the back of the eye. This is the one place in the body where the blood vessels, which course over the retinal surface, may be directly observed. The head of the optic nerve may also be seen through the ophthalmascope and any opacification in the cornea or the lens of the eye, or the vitreous, can be noted by the observer. If a dense cataract or corneal scar is present, or if the vitreous is filled with blood and the retina cannot be observed, an ultrasound examination of the back of the eye may be performed, and at least a rough estimate of whether the retina and choroid are intact and in their proper position can be determined. The principle of ultrasound is similar to the sonar sound wave used by destroyers to detect submerged submarines.

Retinoblastoma and retrolental fibroplasia are two diseases that may affect the retina in children.

Retinoblastoma is a tumor that arises from the retina itself. It has a predilection for young children. Usually it is discovered before the child reaches his first birthday. The tumor is acquired as a dominant hereditary trait. For parents who have had one child with retinoblastoma, there is a 4 to 7 percent chance that any subsequent children will have retinoblastoma. Any person who has been cured of retinoblastoma and who lives to childbearing age should be told that, if they have children, there is a 50 percent chance that the children will be affected by retinoblastoma.

Retinoblastoma is a slow-growing cancer. It is usually enclosed by the sclera and remains in the retina and vitreous for several months before it invades the brain by way of the optic nerve or breaks through the sclera to invade the orbit. If this occurs, death usually results.

The treatment for unilateral retinoblastoma is generally removal of the affected eye. However, retinoblastoma not infrequently affects both eyes. In these cases, radiation may be helpful. Anticancer drugs are also used with some success.

Enucleation has been so successful in treating patients with unilateral retinoblastoma that there are now adults of childbearing age who recovered from the disease but whose children now have retinoblastoma.

Retrolental fibroplasia is the second serious retinal disease of infancy. The disease was unknown prior to the use of high concentrations of oxygen in nurseries for premature babies.

High concentrations of oxygen cause the premature retinal blood vessels to continue to grow and proliferate. As the vessels grow into the vitreous, scar tissue forms and the vitreous contracts, damaging the eye and the retina. Since the cause of retrolental fibroplasia was discovered, the incidence of the disease has declined considerably. Today, pediatricians are careful to limit the amount of oxygen given premature children, and the disease has all but disappeared. Unfortunately, when retrolental fibroplasia does occur, it is bilateral.

The first case of retrolental fibroplasia was reported in 1942. Oxygen was not implicated as the causative factor until 1954. Premature children who were born between 1942 and 1954 are now adults and many of them have severe visual handicaps.

Retinal detachment can occur at any age. However, it is most common in adults and in near-sighted persons. The mechanism underlying retinal detachment is simple. A vacuum causes the retina to adhere closely to the choroid. If wallpaper was held on a wall by a vacuum instead of glue, and a hole was punched in the wallpaper, the vacuum would break and the paper would fall away from the wall. So it is with the elastic retina. Once a hole breaks the vacuum that attaches it to the choroid, the retina begins to peel off the choroid and its elasticity causes it to contract. As contraction increases, so does the rate and amount of separation. Fluid from the vitreous seeps in between the retina and choroid and furthers the separation. Since the retina depends on the vascular choroid for much of its nutrition, separation from its source of supply impairs its function.

Detachment of any portion of the retina results in a corresponding loss of visual field. If the entire retina becomes detached, the eye becomes completely blind. Because of this, when detachment does occur, it is an ophthalmological emergency.

The treatment of retinal detachment is aimed at closing the retinal hole by diathermy or cryothermy applied to the area of the sclera overlying the hole.

Since the retina is elastic and tends to contract when it becomes detached, a sizeable detachment requires that the sclera overlying the area of the detachment be indented inward so that the retina will not have to be stretched back to its original size. For this, a scleral buckling procedure is performed. Sometimes, retina will not have to be stretched back to its original size. For this, a scleral buckling procedure is frequently used. Sometimes, it may be necessary to implant a piece of plastic or other inert material to dent the sclera over the area of the detachment.

Photocoagulation is successful in closing retinal holes that have not

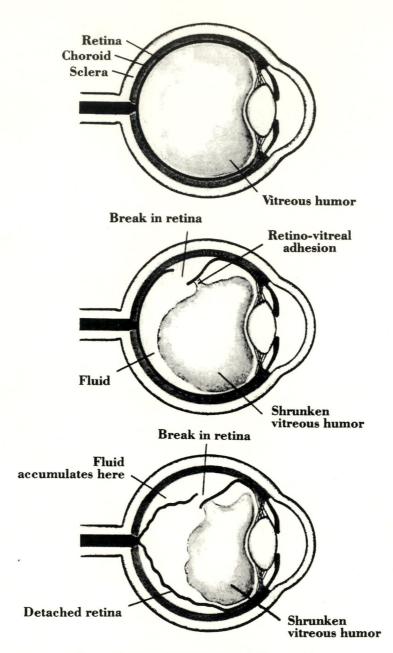

Figure 17. Stages in detachment of the retina.

progressed to retinal detachment. The ophthalmic surgeon performs this operation (which resembles spot welding) under direct visualization. A laser beam is focused upon the area of retina which is still attached around the hole. Several applications of this energy burn the retina around the hole and the resulting scar formation effects a permanent seal between the retina and choroid, thus circumventing retinal detachment.

Patients with myopia (near-sightedness) are more susceptible to retinal detachment than other persons. The myopic eye has grown longer and larger since birth, thereby placing stretch on the retina which does not grow as rapidly as the outer coats of the eye. This stretching tends to make the retina thinner and more vulnerable to tearing. If the near-sighted patient suffers trauma or further retinal degeneration, a hole may appear spontaneously and retinal detachment result.

Occasionally, retinal detachment occurs in patients who have had cataract surgery, especially if vitreous strands have run from the retina to the wound. Vitreous strands tend to contract as time goes on, and when they become firmly attached to the cataract wound, they may pull a hole in the retina.

More rarely, retinal detachments may be found in eyes with malignant melanoma or inflammatory disease of the choroid. The fluid that forms between the choroid and the retina in inflammatory cases elevates the retina. Since no hole exists, the retina will flatten out if the choroidal fluid absorbs spontaneously. On the other hand, if a tumor is present, the detachment will continue to increase as the tumor grows.

There is no pain associated with retinal detachment. The patient will describe lightning flashes and spots of light suddenly bursting in front of his eyes. He will notice a dramatic increase in the number of floaters and generally these floaters will be large, black, annoying spots and streaks. Then a gray curtain slowly covers his field of vision. The ophthalmic surgeon viewing a retinal detachment sees a gray bulge instead of the flat, red reflex of the normal retina. If an early diagnosis of a retinal detachment is made and surgery or laser therapy is performed before it progresses too far, a very high success rate is obtained by a competent retinal surgeon. One or two months of postoperative convalescence are required, and the retinal detachment patient must limit his activity for a period after surgery. If the retinal detachment is not treated, however, blindness will almost certainly result and become permanent. Spontaneous reattachment of the retina is extremely rare.

Senile macular degeneration, a disease of the elderly, results from degeneration of the macular area of the retina. It is usually due to arteriosclerosis or insufficient blood supply through the vessels of the choroid underlying the macular area. In comparison with the circulation in other parts of the retina, the macula is quite avascular. This lack of circulation increases the macula's optical efficiency, but also makes it more vulnerable to vascular disease. Since the macular area depends almost entirely on the choroidal circulation for its meager blood supply, any hemorrhage or occlusion of a blood vessel in the macular area of the choroid almost invariably results in a reduction in the patient's central vision.

The patient with senile macular degeneration complains of difficulty in reading and in seeing things directly ahead. His peripheral vision, however, is not affected, and he is always able to get around and take care of himself. Frequently, a magnifying glass will considerably improve his ability to read by enlarging the words so that their images fall on the surrounding noninvolved retina. There is no good treatment for senile macular degeneration which, unfortunately, tends to be bilateral and tends to progress. However, occasionally, laser is helpful early in the disease. Some people believe dietary supplements of vitamins and minerals are helpful. This is a moot point. Generally, however, the vision does not fall below 20/100 or 20/200 in either eye. An ophthalmologist viewing the macular area sees scarring, increased pigmentation, and, sometimes, hemorrhages and hard exudates.

Hemorrhages of the retina occur rather frequently in two diseases: diabetes and hypertension. The hemorrhages of hypertension are usually flame shaped and superficial. Although they may affect vision at the time, they also may resolve spontaneously with no visual loss. A hypertensive patient may have one or two small hemorrhages that do not involve the macular area and not even be aware of a hemorrhage in his eye.

The diabetic patient usually has more numerous and larger hemorrhages. Because they occupy some of the deeper layers of the retina, the ophthalmologist sees them as blot or dot hemorrhages.

Whereas treating a patient's hypertension results in spontaneous clearing of retinal hemorrhages and helps to prevent further hemorrhaging, treatment of a diabetic's blood sugar level does not guarantee relief from further retinal hemorrhages. In certain diabetic retinopathy cases, laser can be used to seal off any leaking or any potentially weak vessels and can also be used to destroy some of the peripheral retina, which may be effective in reducing the amount of damage caused by the diabetic retinopathy to the central retina. ***Occlusion of the central retinal vein*** is most likely to occur in older or in diabetic persons. Fortunately, this entity is relatively rare. Usually involving only one eye, it results in sudden and painless loss of central vision. The second eye is seldom involved. Through the ophthalmoscope one sees numerous hemorrhages scattered through the entire posterior part of the eye.

All types of treatment for occlusion of the central retinal vein are of little value. Secondary optic atrophy, glaucoma, and retinal degeneration frequently follow the occlusion. However, about one-fifth of patients spontaneously regain at least useful vision.

Occlusion of the central retinal artery is uncommon. It is usually unilateral and occurs in older persons who have arteriosclerosis. The occlusion generally results from a thrombus or plaque, as happens in coronary occlusion. The loss of vision is sudden, painless, and usually complete.

The eye appears to be devoid of blood. The nervehead is pale; the retinal arterioles are collapsed and empty. If the occlusion is complete, visual loss is total and permanent. If, however, the patient is seen within a few minutes after the onset of the occlusion, and if the occlusion is not complete by that time, blood flow may be restored by puncturing the anterior chamber or by rapidly reducing the intraocular pressure with an osmotic agent. A rapid-acting vascular dilator is given at the same time. Rarely is the patient with central retinal artery occlusion seen before most of the vision in the affected eye is lost. The retina survives lack of blood for only a few minutes. Treatment is hopeless if it is delayed for more than a few minutes after the onset of the occlusion.

Retinitis pigmentosa is a genetically determined form of degeneration which begins at the retinal periphery and gradually progresses toward the macular area. The retinal cells are replaced by clumps of pigmented tissue which, to the examining ophthalmologist, look as if a crow had walked across the retina, leaving his muddy footprints.

The onset of retinitis pigmentosa is generally during the teen years. More common in men than in women, it is almost always bilateral.

Nightblindness is one of the first symptoms of retinitis pigmentosa. That is because the peripheral retina, where the rods are located, is involved first. As the disease progresses, the patient usually develops cataracts. Glaucoma is also a frequent complication, as is myopia.

There is no known treatment for retinitis pigmentosa. Gradually the peripheral visual field constricts until, when the patient reaches the age of fifty or sixty years, only three to five degrees of the central field remain. Even so, the central vision in many cases will be sufficient for reading until the patient reaches the age of seventy or eighty years.

Another form of nightblindness, fortunately very rare, results from extreme deprivation of vitamin A. Most cases occur in concentration camps where the diet lacks many vital foods. Vitamin A supplies carotene to the rods which provide night vision. If the diet lacks carotene for any length of time, the available supply is removed from the body, and the rods cannot function. The treatment is, of course, to take vitamin A or to eat foods rich in vitamin A. This is probably the origin of the idea that eating carrots will improve your vision.

The Vitreous

Although the avascular, jellylike vitreous body occupies the greatest volume of the eye and is closely connected to the retina, it is seldom affected by overt disease. However, there is one prevalent vitreous disorder, *vitreous floaters.*

Vitreous floaters are perceived as dust motes, or spots, or tiny undulating streamers that float about, seeming to be in front of the eyes, moving up and down and sideways as the eyes move, disappearing and reappearing. One's first impression is that stragglers from a swarm of insects are dancing in front of one's eyes, that the annoyance is external. This is not so.

The minute particles are in the vitreous itself. They tend to cast shadows on the retina when the light strikes them. The brain perceives the shadows as objects exterior to the eyes. When an ophthalmologist examines the eyes, he can see the particles in the vitreous.

It is probable that some degenerative change causes vitreous floaters. Occasionally, in a hypertensive or a diabetic patient, they result from hemorrhaging into the eye. They may also precede retinal detachment. As the floaters persistently increase in numbers and the detachment progresses, the patient sees large flashes of light. Finally, a curtain seems to descend in front of the eye, blocking out vision. When this occurs, the patient must be seen immediately by an ophthalmologist. However, most vitreous floaters, although annoying, are not serious. They cause no impairment of vision.

One of the recent developments in ophthalmic surgery is the vitrectomy machine. The basic principle of the various vitrectomy machines is the same. A cutting or chopping probe, which is attached to a suction device, is introduced into the vitreous, usually through a small hole cut in the sclera and choroid and retina, just behind the pars plana. The cutting probe acts like a Roto-Rooter® and chops and cuts the vitreous, and if necessary, the lens of the eye, into small particles, which are then irrigated from the eye. Bit by bit, vitreous which is clouded by blood, can be removed and replaced with clear saline solution. This is of great advantage in people who have had a severe vitreous hemorrhage, whether because of diabetes, trauma, hypertension, or other cause. Eyes that have been blinded by vitreous hemorrhages can be restored to sight. The machine is also useful in removing infected vitreous.

Color Blindness

The exact mechanism of color blindness has not, as yet, been elucidated, although it is known that it is a hereditary defect transmitted by the male sex chromosome. The condition occurs almost exclusively in men, the incidence being about 8 percent in men and only 0.4 percent in women. The most common form of color blindness is red-green, which is the inability to distinguish between certain shades of red and green. In some persons, color blindness is complete. The victims can detect no color whatsoever. Consequently, they live in a black and white world.

Occasionally, color blindness occurs in persons who have retinal disease or who have been exposed to toxic materials that damage the cones.

Color blindness is detected by means of various charts and color plates, such as the Ishihara or the HRR pseudo-isochromatic plates.

It is impossible to treat color blindness. The color blind are, of course, handicapped by not being able to distinguish color, and often are limited in their choice of occupation.

QUESTIONS

1. What is the function of the retina?
2. How is the retina nourished?
3. Compare rods and cones.
4. What is a retinoblastoma and what age group is most commonly affected?

5. What causes retrolental fibroplasia?
6. Why does a hole in the retina cause it to detach?
7. What is the most likely result of a retinal detachment if it is not treated?
8. What is the most common form of color blindness?
9. Why are nearsighted people more susceptible to retinal detachment?
10. What is senile macular degeneration?
11. Describe the difference between the typical diabetic hemorrhage and the typical hypertensive hemorrhage.
12. What are vitreous floaters?

Chapter 9

NEURO-OPHTHALMOLOGY:
HOW THE EYES AND BRAIN RELATE

THE optic nerves connect the eyes to the brain. An optic nerve originates in the retina of the eye, extends to the back part of the eye to a sieve-like opening in the sclera. The numerous nerve fibers run through these sieve-like holes in the back of the sclera and then through an opening in the skull bone, the optic foramen.

Just behind the optic foramen, in the brain cavity itself, the two optic nerves (one from each eye) run together at the Chiasm. Here some of the nerve fibers remain on the same side of the brain as the eye of origin and some cross to the other side. In other words, some of the nerve fibers from the right eye go to the right side of the brain and some go to the left. The nerve fibers from the left eye follow the same pattern but in reverse. This arrangement makes the right side of the brain responsible for vision to the left, and the left side of the brain responsible for vision to the right. These fibers continue from the chiasm to the left and right lateral geniculate bodies.

Any injury to the optic nerve before it gets to the optic chiasm results in visual disturbance to one eye only. Any damage to the optic pathways after the nerve fibers have left the chiasm involves both eyes, producing defects that affect one-half of the visual field in each eye. The optic chiasm where the nerve fibers cross is in the form of an X.

The nerve fibers that originated in the retina terminate at the lateral geniculate bodies where they hook up with a new set of nerve fibers that extend back to the occipital lobes of the brain. They act as a relay cable from the lateral geniculate bodies to the visual center in the occipital cortex of the brain (see Figure 5).

The actual visualization of an image and the interpretation of what is visualized occur in the brain itself. Diseases of the optic nerve or those of the brain that affect the optic tracts result in defects in vision or complete loss of sight.

Defects in peripheral vision can be plotted in the visual field. The patient is placed in front of a perimeter which is a device used to plot the visual field. Each eye is measured separately. The eye is fixated on a point at the center of the field and a small object, or light is placed at various locations around the fixation point. The patient responds if he sees the object. Those areas where he does not see the object are blackened out (see Figure 18).

Defects in the field are often very helpful in determining the location of the disease process and often give a good idea as to the cause of the defect.

Among the diseases that affect the optic nerve are inflammation due to viral or bacterial infection and other degenerative diseases, such as *multiple sclerosis.* Familial hereditary primary degeneration can involve the optic nerve spontaneously. Syphilis is another disease that may affect the optic nerve. Glaucoma, poor circulation and trauma may also involve the optic nerve.

Severe infections in the sinuses located near the optic nerve may erode through the surrounding bone and infect the optic nerve. Certain toxic conditions, such as ingestion of methyl alcohol, arsenic, lead, quinine and probably to some extent, tobacco and salicylates, can cause toxic degeneration of the optic nerve.

Any disease process which involves an optic nerve reduces vision in the eye the nerve supplies. Seldom, however, are both optic nerves involved in the same disease process. Glaucoma is an exception.

The chiasm behind the optic foramen may become involved by brain tumors or strokes. *Aneurysms* (ballooning out) of the large blood vessels located near the chiasm can press on the optic nerve fibers in this area. Any involvement of the nerve fibers at or behind the chiasm affects some portion of the vision of both eyes.

Brain tumors behind the lateral geniculate body or aneurysms of large blood vessels in this area can produce pressure on the nerve fibers of the optic tracts, causing similar defects in the visual fields of both eyes. For example, if a brain tumor exerts pressure on the right optic tract before it reaches the occipital lobe, the shape of the defect in the visual field will be approximately the same on the left side of both eyes. This defect is called *homonymous hemianopsia.*

All of these facts make neurologists and neurosurgeons extremely interested in their patients' visual field defects, for frequently visual field studies indicate the type of brain disease present, as well as suggest what part of the brain is affected.

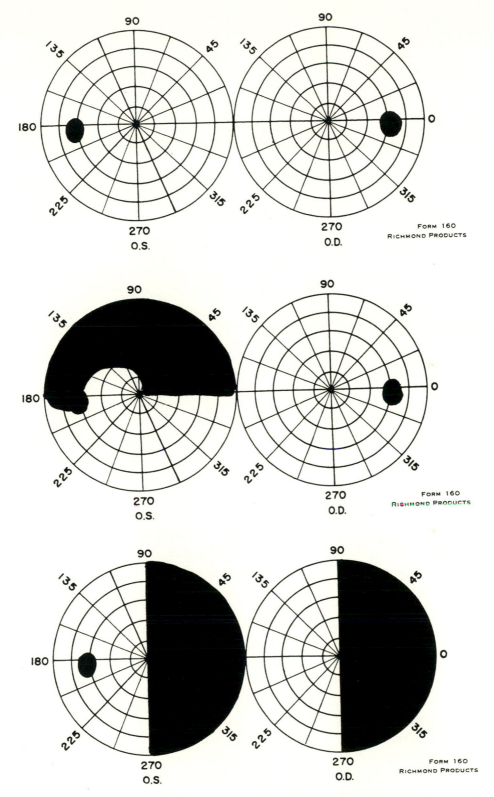

Figure 18. Top. Normal visual field. Center. Typical glaucomatous scotoma left eye (defect in left eye and optic nerve anterior to Chiasm). Bottom. Right homonomus hemianopsia (lesion in brain behind chiasm).

Pupillary reactions and ocular motility are also important in neuro-logical diagnosis. Diseases of the brain may affect the third, fourth, and sixth nerves, which are the motor nerves to the eye. The pupils also provide trustworthy signs of pathologic alterations in the neurological system. There are two dependable tests: the ***pupillary light reflex*** and the ***pupillary accommodative reflex.***

The light reflex test is constriction of the pupils when a bright light is flashed into the eye and their dilation when the light is turned off. The accommodative reflex is constriction of the pupil when the patient looks at a close object after gazing into the distance.

An absent or reduced or hyperactive pupillary reflex is a significant diagnostic sign. Sudden paralysis of one or more of the extraocular muscles which inhibits the accommodative reflex is important in localiz-ing brain disease. One can assume that a motor nerve is involved some-where along its course through the brain, then through the bony openings in the skull to the back of the orbit, then through the orbit to the eye. It is no longer functioning properly. The test indicates the areas most likely involved, either in the brain or in the brain cavity before the nerve reaches the orbit.

The fifth cranial nerve, the principal sensory nerve to the face, to the eyes, and to the orbit, can be attacked by various disease processes. Reduction in its function first causes a slight decrease in sensation in the areas it services. As the disease progresses, definite numbness appears in the face or eyelids and even in the cornea and the eye itself. Sensitivity reactions of the skin around the eye and the reaction of the cornea to the touch of a cotton swab are tests important to neurological evaluation.

Herpes zoster ophthalmacus is a disease that involves the fifth cranial nerve's ophthalmic division. It is caused by a virus similar to the chicken-pox virus, which invades the nerve and causes a very severe rash and breakdown of the skin of the affected side of the forehead, nose, and cheek, which stops exactly at the midline. Therefore, only one eye will be involved and the involved eye may have a severe iritis, corneal changes, and even vitritis and glaucoma. The disease is self-limiting and though there is no way to kill the virus, supportive therapy can be used to protect the eye until the disease burns itself out, although this may take several months.

The seventh cranial nerve, another motor nerve important to the eyes, supplies the orbicularis muscles around the eye, enabling the eyelids to close. It also supplies the various muscles that control facial expression and sends fibers forward to the lacrimal gland, allowing the gland to secrete tears.

If the seventh nerve is damaged, the patient may not be able to close his eyes, nor protect them with tears. This would result in an exposed, dry eye, and the possibility of corneal breakdown and infection would be great.

Brain tumors or diseases of the brain which increase the pressure in the cranial cavity strangulate the veins leaving the inside of the eye through the optic nerve. As a result, blood backs up into the eye, and the nerve becomes congested and swollen. Frequently, the blood vessels break and the blood spattered about the nervehead can be seen with the ophthalmoscope. Termed *papilledema* or *choked disc,* discovering its presence is important in diagnosing and evaluating brain tumors and other diseases causing increased intracranial pressure.

The eye which shows a choked disc or papilledema is usually on the same side as the brain tumor. Slow-growing tumors of the brain may, however, progress insidiously and cause atrophy of the nerve on their side and papilledema on the opposite side, resulting in loss of vision in one eye and a choked disc in the contralateral eye.

Diseases that involve the brain or the blood supply to the brain can cause visual symptoms which are disturbing to the patient. *Scintillating scotomas,* little heat spots, wavy dots, and flashing lights, seen as though they were in front of one eye, frequently occur before a *migraine headache.* Spasms of the blood vessels to one or the other occipital lobe of the brain cause these phenomena which the patient sees as static in the image to the side opposite the affected occipital lobe. When the spasms suddenly end, the vessels dilate, the blood surges forward, and the vessels actually become stretched. This causes the throbbing, pounding one-sided headache experienced by migraine sufferers. Persons who have had migraine for a time know that, if they take cafergot (a mixture of caffeine and ergotamine) when they first see the scintillating scotomas, the headache will be aborted before the pain begins. Other medications are also helpful.

Patients who have diseases of the blood vessels supplying the brain often find that a sudden change in vision is the first hint that something is wrong. They experience double vision or sudden disappearance of part of their visual field. These ocular changes may be permanent if the person has had a severe stroke, or they may be transient when the reduction in the flow of blood to the brain is temporary and returns to normal in a short time. To illustrate: when an airplane pilot pulls out of a dive, the blood suddenly flows from the brain to the lower part of his body, producing the sensation of *blacking out*. Vision is the first faculty to black out.

When an ophthalmologist examines a person's eyes, not only does he obtain information as to the patient's general health but also his examination often discloses that a neurological disease exists.

QUESTIONS

1. Trace the course of the visual impulse originating on the left side of the left eye all the way back to the occipital lobe.
2. What side of the brain is responsible for vision to the patient's right?
3. Will damage to an optic pathway behind the chiasm involve the vision in one eye or in both?
4. List some conditions which may cause loss of function of the optic nerve.
5. How can a visual field be helpful in diagnosing a brain tumor?
6. Describe the pupillary reflexes and how they might be helpful to a neurosurgeon.
7. What is the nerve that supplies the sensation to the face?
8. If the lids of one eye cannot be closed, what nerve is probably responsible?
9. Describe a choked disc.
10. What is a scintillating scotoma?
11. What causes a pilot to black out?
12. List the cranial nerves of particular interest to the ophthalmologist.

Chapter 10

STRABISMUS: THE WANDERING EYE

THERE are certain advantages and certain problems in possessing two eyes. The most obvious advantage is that, if something happens to one eye, the other eye will still enable one to see. Two eyes functioning together enhance depth perception and give the regarded image a third dimension that cannot be wholly achieved by only one eye.

The dilemma facing the gunnery officer of a destroyer illustrates the problem encountered by two eyes which have to work together. The officer has a cannon in the bow and a cannon in the stern. He plans to fire a broadside at an object off his starboard side. If the object is a number of miles away, shots from the two cannons can be approximately parallel and, if they are lined directly upon the enemy vessel, both shells will hit the target at approximately the same place. If, however, the object is much closer, perhaps just a few hundred yards off the side, the two cannons must be pointed in toward each other closer and closer so that both line up on the enemy vessel.

Our two eyes have a similar problem. If the regarded object is far away, alignment of the two eyes must be approximately parallel if the observed image is to fall on the macular area of each eye. If, however, one is looking at something close, e.g. trying to thread a needle or read the print in a telephone directory, the two eyes have to turn in toward each other if the image is to fall on the macular area of each eye.

Turning of the eyes toward each other is called *convergence*. When the eyes point out toward an object in the far distance, they parallel each other. This action, called *divergence,* describes their transition from pointing toward each other to resuming their practically parallel position. It is also possible to have one eye that points higher than the other. If the two eyes are not trained on the same object their owner will actually perceive two different objects. One eye will see the object of regard; the second eye will be pointing toward some other spot in the visual field. If both eyes are functioning normally, the result is double vision. One image will fall on the macula of the right eye and the other image on the macula of the left eye.

If John's face appears on the right macula and Susan's face on the left, it is difficult to decide whether one sees John or Susan because the brain will superimpose the image of each face, and the result will be double vision (***diplopia***). This considerable confusion in one's brain is extremely annoying.

The phenomenon of double vision occurs most often in very young children who adapt easily to almost any situation. A child with double vision tends to favor one eye over the other. He will suppress (disregard) the image from the unfavored eye and will see only one face, not the superimposed faces. The price he pays will be the sacrifice of his ability to fuse images and acquire a three-dimensional picture.

If this process continues for a long time, the brain will forget the unfavored eye, the one with the suppressed vision. Gradually, this eye will become ignored and, as time goes on, the condition will become irreversible. This condition is called ***amblyopia ex anopsia,*** and the eye affected with this disorder will never see well during the remainder of the victim's life, even if the good eye becomes blind.

About 5 percent of children have strabismus, a condition that demands treatment during childhood, the earlier the better.

The orbit of the eye is, to continue the destroyer analogy, the turret of the eye. Six extraocular muscles move the eye in the orbit. They are (1) the medial rectus which pulls the eye in toward the nose, (2) the lateral rectus which pulls the eye away from the nose, (3) the superior rectus which primarily elevates the eye, (4) the inferior rectus whose main function is to depress the eye.

These four rectus muscles originate at the back of the bony orbit in a little circle surrounding the optic nerve. This circle, called the annulus of Zinn after the ubiquitous scientist, must not be confused with the zonules of Zinn, the little "guy wires" that suspend the lens inside the eye.

The four rectus muscles run forward to insert into the tough sclera of the eye. The superior rectus inserts superiorly, the medial rectus toward the inside, the lateral rectus toward the outside, and the inferior rectus below. When the medial rectus contracts, the lateral rectus must relax. When the inferior rectus contracts, the superior rectus relaxes.

The two remaining extraocular muscles are (5) the superior oblique and (6) the inferior oblique. The oblique muscles differ from the rectus muscles because they tend to angle in from the nasal side of the orbit and attach obliquely to the sclera. Although the primary function of the oblique muscles is to rotate the eye in its socket, their secondary function is to elevate and depress the eye.

Innervation of these six extraocular muscles comes from the third, fourth, and sixth cranial nerves. The third cranial nerve innervates the medial, superior and inferior rectus muscles as well as the inferior oblique muscle. It is the same nerve that supplies the ciliary muscle with its accommodative power.

The sixth cranial nerve supplies the lateral rectus muscle and is solely responsible for the abduction of the eye. The fourth cranial nerve innervates the superior oblique muscle.

Of the three cranial nerves controlling ocular movements, the third cranial nerve is the most important, for it effects accommodation as well as contraction of the medial rectus to cause the eyes to converge. Because of this, there is a definite relationship between a person's ability to accommodate and to converge. Usually, if an individual tends to over-accommodate, he will tend to overconverge and align his eyes at a point much closer to his face than the object actually is located. This is the mechanism that most frequently causes crossing of the eyes.

Coordination of the eyes and their ability to work together develop from about the age of five or six weeks to about the age of six months. The sensory pattern of the eyes is not completely fixed until about the age of six or seven years. During this interval, it is capable of adjusting to new mechanical alignments. This is why the earlier the wandering eye is spotted, the easier it is to correct the condition and obtain a good functional result. Perfect binocular alignment of the eyes in all positions of gaze and good fusion of vision is the ideal objective of correction, and the longer one eye deviates and its vision is suppressed, the more difficult it is to correct the problem and prevent amblyopia.

The second most common cause of strabismus is a hereditary tendency for the eyes to turn in or out at an early age. Unless this condition is corrected during the first few years of life, amblyopia generally occurs, and the child, like his forbears, goes through life with one wandering, lazy, amblyopic eye. The family history is, therefore, an essential element of the examination of a child with strabismus.

The amount of deviation is measured with prisms and recorded. It is important to determine the refractive error under cycloplegia because the use of atropine, Cyclogyl, or other cycloplegic drops abolishes the accommodative mechanism, thereby allowing exact determination of the amount of farsightedness or nearsightedness. Most children whose eyes turn in are quite farsighted which, usually, is the reason their eyes turn in; to look at a close object, a farsighted person has to accommodate considerably more than a nearsighted or normal sighted individual. Overaccommodation overstimulates the third cranial nerve and causes the medial rectus muscles to overconverge and align at a point far closer to the child's face than is the object he is actually looking at.

Interestingly, the eyes of many nearsighted children tend to diverge because it is not necessary to accommodate to see something close. The result is that one eye lines up on something close and the other eye drifts out.

After the ophthalmologist has made a diagnosis of strabismus, he has a number of ways in which he can correct the condition. Glasses are his first and, perhaps, most important tool. If the problem is excessive accommodation in a farsighted child, the prescription of farsighted glasses or even bifocals may solve the problem (if the child wears them).

Generally, these children will wear their glasses happily because the glasses reduce the diplopia they have been experiencing. It is now possible to use the eyes together to achieve fusion and make possible using the eyes together to achieve fusion and three-dimensional vision, which is pleasant.

Another correction possibility for young individuals is to use eyedrops (such as phospholine iodide) which cause overaccommodation and force the ciliary muscle to contract by itself without any innervation from the third nerve. The effect is to make the child more nearsighted. Conquering overaccommodation solves the problem of overconvergence that causes inturning of the eyes, thereby stabilizing normal alignment of the eyes. Unfortunately, these drops tend to produce side-effects and cannot be used over a long period. Even so, eyedrops can be useful in a very young child.

If the deviation of his eye is not too great, a child may benefit from eye exercises under the supervision of an *orthoptic technician,* a trained professional who has specialized in the exercises designed to straighten eyes and improve fusion.

If glasses, eyedrops, and orthoptic exercises are not sufficiently effective, eye muscle surgery may be indicated. The surgery is based on the principle of strengthening or weakening the action of an involved muscle. Removing a muscle (or muscles) from its attachment to the sclera of the eye and moving it back behind the area of its original insertion and reinserting it into the sclera by means of small sutures will weaken the muscle. The operation is performed through the conjunctiva which is then closed with small sutures. The child may be hospitalized. Or the surgery may be done on an outpatient basis.

The strengthening operation can be done separately or at the same time as the weakening procedure. An incision is made through the conjunctiva, the desired muscle is isolated and removed from its scleral attachment. A section (generally from three to seven millimeters) of the muscle itself is removed and the remaining muscle is reattached to its original insertion. The shorter muscle working over the same distance produces more forceful contractions and causes a greater action on the movement of the eye.

The horizontal deviations are the most common deviations of the eyes, causing inturning or outturning of the eyes in relation to each other. Inturning is called *esotropia;* outturning is called *exotropia.*

It is also possible for one eye to point higher than the other. In this case, the higher eye is said to have *hypertropia* although, actually, its muscles may not be responsible. The opposite eye, which actually is pointing down, may be the affected eye. This is called *hypotropia.* (However, for simplification, we seldom speak of hypotropia. Usually the higher eye is selected and the case is called one of hypertropia.)

Another form of strabismus or deviation of the eyes occurs in older persons who have had perfectly normal binocular vision all their lives. Suddenly, or slowly, they develop double vision, an extremely annoying condition which they had never before experienced. Adults are not as adaptable as children. They can no longer suppress the image in one eye to avoid double vision. This condition can be treated simply by covering or occluding one eye or the other. However, it is most important to investigate the underlying cause, which may be a hemorrhage into the brain where one of the nerves supplying an extraocular muscle originates and, therefore, may be the sign of a stroke.

A brain tumor or other diseases of the brain can affect one or more of the extraocular muscles, reducing or obliterating its function and paralyzing the muscles it supplies. In addition, the pupillary and accommodation reflexes which come to the eye through the third nerve may be involved simultaneously. For these reasons, a neurosurgeon or neurologist routinely examines the motility of the eyes, the reaction of the pupils, and the ability of the patient to accommodate.

Usually, a paretic strabismus in an adult is extremely difficult to treat unless the underlying cause is treated. Frequently, if the eye disorder is secondary to a minor stroke, diabetes, or high blood pressure, simply treating the underlying condition will gradually improve the alignment of the eyes and cause the diplopia to recede.

Exercises, surgery, the use of eyedrops or regular glasses usually give unsatisfactory results in these cases. More often, symptomatic improvement can be obtained by placing prisms in the patient's glasses or by occluding one eye. Amblyopia seldom occurs in older individuals. This is a mixed blessing, however, for the diplopia continues as long as the eyes are out of alignment and while both eyes are open.

QUESTIONS

1. What are some of the advantages of having two eyes?
2. What is convergence?
3. What is double vision and why may double vision occur?
4. What is amblyopia ex anopsia?
5. What muscle pulls the eye in toward the nose?
6. What is the most important nerve as far as the extraocular muscles are concerned?
7. When do we learn to use our eyes together?
8. Why is it important to determine the refractive error in considering strabismus?
9. Who is an orthoptic technician?
10. How can we surgically weaken a muscle, and how can we surgically strengthen a muscle?
11. What is meant by paretic strabismus?
12. What conditions may cause paretic strabismus?

Chapter 11

EYE CHANGES ASSOCIATED
WITH GENERAL DISEASE

MANY diseases which affect the entire body frequently are revealed in the eye at an early stage, making possible the diagnosis of a generalized disease process by examining the eyes.

The eye is a window to the vascular system of the body. By using an ophthalmoscope, a physician can visualize the retinal arteries and veins which often manifest changes that are also present in the blood vessels throughout the body. Thus the retinal blood vessels of patients with high blood pressure, diabetes, endocrine disorders, or hardening of the arteries will show characteristic changes.

Other systemic diseases will affect the clarity of the lens, the amount of tear formation, the eye muscles, and so on. The ophthalmologist frequently detects a general disease process and refers a patient to the appropriate physician for further diagnostic procedures and treatment.

Arteriosclerosis (hardening of the arteries), the most common change in the arterioles, is associated with the aging process. Arteriosclerotic changes in the eye are primarily limited to the arteries. Many individuals show arteriosclerosis after they reach middle age. Persons who have hypertension or diabetes, as well as some individuals with no associated disease, may develop these changes earlier.

The basic problem in arteriosclerosis is thickening of the walls of the blood vessels, compressing the blood column and making it smaller and smaller. As the sclerosis progresses, the walls of the arteries become hard. It is easy to see the sclerotic walls of the blood vessels with the ophthalmoscope.

Occasionally blood vessels will become plugged. If this happens to the main artery entering through the optic nerve, the blood supply to the retina is shut off. This disaster, called *occlusion of the central retinal artery*, results in sudden, almost complete, blindness for which there is no adequate treatment.

If, after it has entered the eye and is coursing over the retina, one of the branches of the central retinal artery becomes occluded, the retinal tissue it supplied will die and cause a partial defect in the field of vision. The defect will correspond to the area of the retina that has been deprived of its blood supply.

A similar sclerotic process can occur in the veins of the retina. When a sclerotic vein becomes totally or partially occluded, the increased pressure caused by the back-up of venous blood behind the area of the occlusion first weakens and then breaks through the wall. Hemorrhage results. *Occlusion of a retinal vein* is usually associated with large retinal hemorrhages which are easily seen with the ophthalmoscope. Occlusion of a retinal artery collapses the vessels behind the clot and, because the wall of an artery is much stronger than the wall of a vein, there is no break. All that the ophthalmoscope shows is pallor and loss of the normal pink color of the blood vessel and retina beyond the area of occlusion.

Hypertension

Persons who have high blood pressure (hypertension) show characteristic changes in their retinal arteries. Spasms or narrowing of the arterial walls are the earliest changes. Perhaps these changes actually provoke hypertension in some individuals, because it takes a higher pressure to force the same amount of blood through smaller vessels.

The muscular walls of the arterial blood vessels contract, narrowing the vessels and forcing the heart to work harder to push blood at a higher pressure through the narrowed arteries. This so-called *essential hypertension* occurs for no apparent reason. As the arterial spasms continue and sclerotic thickening occurs in the vessel walls, the pressure may become so high that, like an old garden hose, the vessels break and spray red blood around the posterior portion of the eye.

The typical *flame shape* of these hemorrhages results from the distribution of the arterial system in the retina. The retinal arterioles run on the inner surface of the retina. At this level, the nerve fibers course toward the optic nervehead in sheets or bundles. When the blood vessel breaks, the blood fans out along the nerve fibers and causes a hemorrhage that looks like a flame, or as if the retina had received one sideways brush stroke of red paint. In more severe hypertension, the optic nerve may become edematous and surrounded by flame-shaped hemorrhages.

Cotton-wool exudates (discharges) occur here and there in retinas in which the blood supply has been impaired. In such cases, the partially damaged vessel walls leak fluid, but not the larger red blood cells, into the retina.

Severe hypertension may result in the rupture of a retinal arteriole and a henorrhage into the retinal tissue and occasionally even into the vitreous body. If this occurs, vision may be damaged, either temporarily or permanently.

If hypertension is diagnosed early, it usually can be controlled medically; the retinal changes, if they have not progressed to the severe later stages, are readily reversible. The spastic blood vessels will return to normal size; any small hemorrhages will absorb without damage to the eye; the cotton-wool patches will absorb and the edematous nerve will return to normal.

One severe form of hypertensive retinopathy occurs in pregnant women toward the time of delivery. For no apparent reason, their blood pressure will suddenly shoot with extreme rapidity to a high level. All the changes found in hypertensive retinopathy may occur in just a few days. Simply terminating the pregnancy and delivering the baby, if necessary by Caesarean section, will correct this situation which, fortunately, is rare. When it does occur during pregnancy, it is a serious threat to the mother's life. The condition is called *eclampsia.*

Diabetes Mellitus

Diabetes is a common disease that is due to numerous complex factors. Simply, the cause is the failure of the pancreas to produce enough insulin to metabolize the blood sugar properly. Eventually diabetes involves blood vessels everywhere in the body, but its most obvious effect is on the eyes and the kidneys.

Diabetic retinopathy seldom occurs in the diabetic patient until the disorder has existed for at least five years. Some patients with a history of diabetes for several decades show absolutely no signs of diabetic retinopathy. It is not unusual for persons who are afflicted with diabetes during childhood or adolescence to manifest more severe forms of diabetic retinopathy during their adulthood than those who developed milder forms of diabetes later in life.

Probably the most characteristic early change in the retinal blood vessels of diabetic patients is a *microaneurysm.* The small ballooning out of the wall of a capillary, which normally is virtually invisible, becomes visible during an ophthalmoscopic examination. The ophthalmologist can see the dilated sac of pooled blood on the otherwise invisible vessel; to him, the microaneurysm looks like a small cherry or a small cluster of cherries in an apparently avascular portion of the retina. The dilatation is on the venous side of the capillary network. Diabetes generally affects the veins more severely than the arterioles.

After the microaneurysms appear, *hard* discharges that resemble tiny drops of wax are seen here and there on the retinal surface. Next, *blot* or *dot hemorrhages* become scattered over the retina. These hemorrhages look like blots because they occur in the deeper layers of the retina (in contrast to flame-shaped hypertensive hemorrhages) where the more compact nerve tissue allows the blood to spread only a little.

In the final stages of diabetic retinopathy, enormous retinal and preretinal hemorrhages occur. Hemorrhages into the vitreous make that structure opaque. Often, the retina is not visible; if it is, one will discover the presence of scar formation. The shrinking scar tissue pulls on the retinal surface. Ultimately, the retina tears. A retinal detachment ensues.

In an attempt to maintain the blood supply to the retina, new blood vessels form, proliferate, and course about the nervehead and out onto the surface of the retina. Since these blood vessels are extremely fragile, they break easily and cause more hemorrhaging which results in additional scar formation and further deterioration inside the eye. At last the retina detaches completely. The eye is blind.

The therapy for diabetic retinopathy is unsatisfactory at best. Many different treatments have been tried. Some physicians feel that maintaining excellent control of the diabetes tends to delay or prevent serious retinal consequences. However, many patients under excellent diabetic control have developed diabetic retinopathy and become blind.

Laser *Photocoagulation* (burning with light) of a leaking blood vessel gives satisfactory results in carefully selected cases. Vitrectomy surgery can be performed on diabetics who have hemorrhaged into the vitreous. This process enables the retinal surgeon to remove the blood and the vitreous together, substituting clear saline solution for the murky, bloody vitreous contents. Laser can also be used to obliterate peripheral areas of the retina, reducing the area requiring a blood supply. This often causes a remission of the disease process in the central retina.

Any treatment of diabetic retinopathy is very difficult to evaluate because the disease tends to have remissions and exacerbations. Microaneurysms may disappear for no apparent reason. Hemorrhages may disappear spontaneously. The condition may suddenly improve for reasons unknown. On the other hand, an almost normal-appearing diabetic eye may, over a short period, progress through all the stages of diabetic retinopathy.

Cataract formation, as well as diabetic retinopathy, occurs frequently in diabetic patients. Often an opacity forms in the posterior portion of the lens in the very center where it greatly reduces vision. Typical senile cataracts may also appear in diabetic patients, often at a relatively early age.

Paralysis of one or more extraocular muscle is not unusual in diabetics, nor is optic neuritis or optic atrophy. The incidence of these conditions is higher in diabetic patients than in the general population.

Sudden changes in refraction occur in diabetics. As the bloodsugar level fluctuates so does the refractive status, often by as much as several diopters. These changes are due to variations in the hydration of the lens. If any of his patients show frequent fluctuations in refraction, the ophthalmologist should suspect the presence of diabetes.

Thyrotoxicosis

Persons who have disturbances of the thyroid gland frequently manifest characteristic eye changes. *Lid lag* is the most common symptom. As the patient looks from up to down, the eyelid, instead of following the downward course in a smooth, normal pattern, tends to remain in the wide-open position for an instant or two. Then, suddenly, almost as if it were just getting the signal, the eyelid will move downward to cover the top of the eye. This immediately suggests the presence of an incipient hyperthyroid problem.

Often, in persons with severe hyperthyroidism, the eyes bulge forward and give a wide-open, fixed gaze appearance. Often, too, these patients develop alterations in their eye movements because of weakness of the eye muscles. Especially affected is convergence. It becomes more and more difficult to focus both eyes on reading material. Double vision and, perhaps, headaches result.

Treatment of hyperthyroidism generally brings about some improvement in the eye findings. However, especially if the hyperthyroidism is quite severe, the eyes protrude and the protrusion may be permanent. The condition is called *proptosis*.

Protuberant eyes are more exposed and dry more rapidly than normal. Any dust or dirt in the air is more likely to fall on the exposed eye. Patients with the proptosis of hyperthyroidism complain of dry, burning, irritated eyes. Frequent use of lubricating eyedrops will help alleviate the irritation. Occasionally, however, the eyelids must be partially closed by a surgical procedure in order to protect the eyes.

Some common infectious diseases that may involve the eyes are tuberculosis, syphilis, measles, smallpox, herpes simplex and herpes zoster (shingles). Reactions to smallpox vaccine may also involve the eyes.

Tuberculosis may cause iritis or chorioretinitis. It may also cause scleritis or episcleritis (inflammation of the sclera). Tuberculosis may also affect the ocular blood vessels, causing retinal hemorrhages. Active tuberculosis can migrate into the interior of the eye and produce tuberculous endophthalmitis, disintegrating the entire eye and turning it into a bag of pus.

Syphilis is a much more subtle disease. It may be present congenitally from the mother and result in ***Hutchinson's*** famous ***triad*** of saddle nose, deafness, and notched incisor teeth, along with interstitial keratitis.

A common eye lesion in syphilis is interstitial keratitis, a haziness of the deep stromal layers of the cornea. Frequently associated with this form of keratitis are vascularization of the cornea and lowgrade chronic iritis. Corneal transplantation may be required to restore useful vision.

Acquired syphilis may cause chorioretinitis and degeneration of the retina, as well as interstitial keratitis, later in life.

Various changes in the way the pupil reacts to light are characteristic of syphilis. Known as the ***Argyll Robertson pupil,*** the changes assist in diagnosing syphilis.

Herpes simplex is a viral disease manifested most often as a ***cold sore*** on the lips. However, if a cold sore attacks the cornea, the result is ***herpetic keratitis.*** This entity is described in the chapter on the cornea.

Herpes zoster (shingles) ophthalmicus is caused by invasion of the shingles virus into the nucleus of the fifth cranial nerve, the nerve that supplies the middle portion of the face from the forehead to the cheek and controls all sensation in the eye, the eyelids, and the surrounding tissues. The skin on the involved side of the face breaks down and forms blisters. If the eye becomes involved, keratitis, iritis, and occasionally, optic neuritis occur. In most cases, the condition clears by itself. To protect the eye, such supportive medications as topical antibiotics and corticosteroids may be needed.

If **German measles** (rubella) infects a woman during the first trimester of pregnancy, it generally causes a number of congenital anomalies in the child, including several serious ocular disorders. Rubella-infected children may be born with bilateral cataracts, **nystagmus** (oscillating eyes), **microphthalmos** (extremely small, nonfunctioning eyes), and strabismus.

Cataract surgery usually is delayed until the child is at least two years of age. Surgery could activate the live rubella virus still present in the ocular tissues during the child's early life and cause complete loss of the eye.

Measles (rubeola) may produce acute conjunctivitis during its course. Occasionally, keratitis results.

Aids patients may have devastating eye infections.

Certain vitamins and drugs can cause ocular complications. **Hypovitamin A** (lack of vitamin A) may result in night blindness. Vitamin A is essential to the formation of visual purple in the retina, and visual purple is essential to the proper function of the rod cells. If vitamin A levels in the body become extremely low, visual purple will not function properly; the rods will not work, and night blindness ensues.

Proper metabolism of the cornea also depends on vitamin A. If vitamin A is long absent from the diet, the cornea becomes dry and hazy, and its epithelium will slough off. As corneal sensitivity decreases, the cornea's defense against bacteria lessens. The infected corneal ulcers that appear scar the cornea. Severe visual loss may result.

Fortunately, vitamin A deficiency is seldom seen in the Western World. It is more prevalent in the malnourished populations of Asia and Africa.

The obvious treatment for lack of vitamin A is administration of vitamin A, generally intramuscularly at first. If corneal scarring has not occurred, this therapy produces rapid return of normal night vision as well as corneal clearing.

It is also possible to get too much vitamin A. This fat-soluble vitamin cannot be excreted from the body at a rapid rate. If a health faddist takes too much vitamin A, various tissues, such as the skin and the sclera, will turn yellow. Too much vitamin A can also affect the brain, causing bilateral papilledema. Conceivably, such patients could die of brain damage.

Anticholinergics (atropine and related drugs) are given systemically for various gastrointestinal disorders. Ophthalmologists also use these preparations topically to dilate the pupil and paralyze the ciliary body during refraction. In large doses, these drugs paralyze accommodation which causes dilatation of the pupil and blurring of vision. More dangerous, if the patient who takes these drugs has an anterior chamber with a narrow angle, is the possibility of an acute attack of glaucoma. Dilatation of the pupil causes the iris to block the angle and the ocular drainage system. Occasionally, a case of acute glaucoma occurs in hospitals after a patient has been given anticholinergic drugs during surgery.

Oral Contraceptives

Oral contraceptives may occasionally precipitate ophthalmic vascular occlusive disease or damage the optic nerve. Occurrences of both of these conditions in patients on oral contraceptives have been documented. However, it seems likely that oral contraceptives are safe when taken by normal healthy women with no history of vascular disease.

Corticosteroids are used widely in medicine both systemically and, in ophthalmology and dermatology, topically. In certain susceptible persons, systemic corticosteroids can cause, over a period of time, increased intraocular pressure, which eventually leads to glaucoma.

Corticosteroids can worsen episodes of fungal keratitis and herpes simplex keratitis. Long-term use of these preparations often stimulates the development of posterior subcapsular cataracts. Usually the cataracts are mild and cause little decrease in vision, but they can be a significant complication of long-term corticosteroid therapy.

Digitalis in high doses may cause blurred vision and disturbed color sensation. Usually, when the digitalis dose is lowered, these symptoms clear. Patients suffering from digitalis intoxication may notice that objects appear yellow or green or, sometimes, snowy white.

Oxygen

Any high concentration of oxygen may cause transient visual blurring in adults. An occasional patient with inactive retrobulbar neuritis may suffer almost complete loss of the visual field following the administration of oxygen.

The most serious consequence of oxygen administration occurs in premature infants. If they receive high concentrations of oxygen for a prolonged period, *retrolental fibroplasia* may affect the eyes. This tragedy is described in the chapter on the retina.

QUESTIONS

1. How can arteriosclerosis affect the eyes?
2. How can hypertension affect the eyes?
3. Describe some eye changes associated with diabetes.
4. What is a microaneurysm?
5. What is photocoagulation?
6. Give some eye problems associated with thyroid disorders.
7. What is interstitial keratitis and what causes it?
8. How can German measles affect an unborn baby's eyes?
9. What eye changes occur under conditions of extreme vitamin A deprivation?
10. What stomach medicines can precipitate an acute closed-angle attack of glaucoma?
11. What eye problems can be caused by corticosteroids?
12. What complaints might a patient on an overdose of digitalis have in regard to his eyes?
13. What is the most serious complication of oxygen therapy in infants?

Chapter 12

INJURIES

INJURIES to the eyes are common even with the extensive use of industrial safety goggles and widespread publicity emphasizing protection of the eyes. A corneal *foreign body* or speck in the eye is the most common eye injury. A small piece of a foreign substance, a cinder, perhaps, becomes imbedded in the cornea or in the conjunctiva of the upper or lower eyelid, causing a scratchy sensation and irritation.

Usually a foreign body can be removed from the conjunctiva by irrigation with water or with a cotton tipped applicator without the help of a physician. If the foreign body is imbedded in the corneal epithelium or in deeper corneal tissues, local anesthesia (instillation of a drop of Ophthaine® or tetracaine) is required before the foreign body can be easily removed with a sharp, knifelike instrument called a corneal spud. After removal of the foreign body, the small pit or crater in the corneal surface will be closed rapidly by the surrounding epithelium growing into the area of the defect.

To promote rapid healing, antibiotic eyedrops and a patch should be applied to the eye. The eye patch will immobilize the eyelids and decrease the friction between the eyelids and the epithelial surface, allowing the epithelium to grow more rapidly. A bandage contact lens may be used instead of the patch.

A corneal abrasion caused by a foreign body will usually heal in twenty-four to forty-eight hours. When a twig, a fingernail, or a piece of paper or some other object scratches the surface of the cornea, a corneal abrasion results. It, too, will heal rapidly if an antibiotic solution is instilled and the eye is patched.

Occasionally, however, linear corneal abrasions recur weeks or months after the healing of the original injury. Indeed, there may be several recurrences over a period of years. The probable cause is failure of the epithelial cells to become adequately reattached to the underlying Bowman's membrane during the initial healing. A foreign body sensation and discomfort warn of the recurrence. Treatment consists of repatching the eye and allowing the abrasion to reheal. The use of a lubricating ointment at bedtime may also be useful in preventing reoccurrences.

Actinic or *ultraviolet radiation keratitis* is another type of injury that can cause damage to the corneal epithelium. It is due to prolonged exposure to a sun lamp, a welding arc, or to the direct rays of the sun. The actinic radiation causes the epithelium to break down, usually within six to twelve hours after exposure to the ultraviolet light. Many dotlike spots cover the corneal surface after it is stained with fluorescein. The involved areas have a punctate, moth-eaten appearance. To the observing ophthalmologist, the cornea looks as if it had been peppered with microscopic buckshot.

An ultraviolet burn is treated with antibiotic eyedrops and the eye is patched for twenty-four to forty-eight hours. Although actinic keratitis is very uncomfortable, it seldom causes permanent damage to the eye.

Flash burns of the eye resemble ultraviolet keratitis. **Chemical burns** of the eye can be extremely serious. Lye causes the most dangerous of common ocular chemical burns because its progressive chemical reaction first destroys the protein of the corneal epithelium, then of Bowman's membrane, and finally, the corneal stroma. Lye burns are frequently bilateral and often result in extreme scarring of both corneas and of the conjunctiva. Shrinkage of the conjunctiva causes the eyelashes to roll in and further irritate the surface of the eye. Eyes burned with lye are difficult to graft (corneal transplant) successfully.

Any potent industrial chemical (acids, alkalis, strong salt solutions, cleaning compounds) can also cause chemical burns of the eyes.

Water is the best and most important treatment for any ocular chemical burn. As soon as the chemical comes in contact with the eye, the eye should be immediately, vigorously, and copiously irrigated with water. Anyone who gets a chemical in his eye should put his head under the nearest faucet, turn on the water and let it run over the eye for five to ten minutes. Any of the chemical removed immediately may not damage the eye; any that is allowed to remain will cause prolonged and extensive damage.

Many foreign bodies in the eye remain in the superficial cornea. A foreign body from a rapidly moving object (a piece of drill bit, bb pellets, the end of a stick or dart) can penetrate the cornea or sclera and become lodged in the interior of the eye.

An occasional foreign body travels directly through the eye, penetrating the cornea or sclera on its way in, penetrating the sclera at the back of the eye, and finally, lodging in the orbit or the bony wall of the orbit. If the foreign body remains lodged in the eye, the ophthalmologist must attempt to remove it. Only an inert object (for example, glass and some plastics) can occasionally be left in the eye without causing further damage.

If the foreign body is magnetic, a magnet can often be used to pull it through an incision in the sclera, choroid, and retina. The retina surrounding the incision is cauterized so that retinal detachment will not occur. A nonmagnetic foreign body is difficult to remove. Sometimes, a foreign body in the anterior portion of the eye can be removed by opening the anterior chamber and extracting the object under direct visualization. However, if a nonmagnetic foreign body is in the back of the eye and cannot be directly visualized, successful removal is very difficult and the results are often poor.

Penetrating foreign bodies are extremely serious. Frequently, they cause secondary damage to the eye, such as cataract, glaucoma, retinal detachment, and disastrous intraocular infection.

When the surface of the eye is cut through and through by some sharp instrument or tool (a knife, an arrow, a screwdriver) the injury is called *laceration of the globe.* Lacerations usually occur in the cornea. If the lacerations involve the central cornea, the resulting scar will cause considerable loss of vision. Eventually, in these cases, a corneal transplant may successfully restore vision. Secondary complications often follow lacerations of the globe. Cataract and retinal detachment are among the complications.

Any individual with a lacerated globe or a penetrating foreign body in the eye should see an ophthalmologist immediately. In the meantime, the eye should be patched. To prevent further damage, the eye should never be touched or examined by anyone other than an ophthalmologist.

A blunt blow to the eye seldom ruptures the globe. It does, however, cause contusion of the globe which resembles a bruise elsewhere in the body. The blow may produce a shock wave that passes across the contents of the eye and causes damage to the retina. If retinal hemorrhages and edema in the macular area follow the injury, there may be rapid loss of vision. Retinal hemorrhage and macular edema that are not severe usually clear and the patient's vision improves considerably.

Occasionally, blunt trauma to the eye breaks a blood vessel in the iris. The resulting bleeding into the anterior chamber is called *hyphema.*

Hyphema is treated by rest to prevent further hemorrhaging. In these cases, it is essential to prevent a rise in the intraocular pressure while the clot occupies the anterior chamber and blocks the trabecular meshwork at the angle. This is a type of glaucoma, which may force the iron pigment from the blood into the cornea, resulting in a tattooed cornea.

If the eye is struck vigorously with a blunt object (for example, a human fist), the floor of the orbit, which is composed of extremely thin bone, may break. This injury, called a *blowout fracture,* may occur concurrently with contusion of the globe, or it may occur when the globe is only slightly injured. A blowout fracture displaces the contents of the orbit through the orbital floor and into the maxillary sinus which lies directly below. If the displacement includes the inferior rectus muscle or the inferior oblique muscle, motion of the eye is limited and pain accompanies each movement. In addition, the eye may have an obvious sunken appearance and lack the prominence of the fellow eye.

To repair the defect in the floor of the orbit, a plastic plate may be placed above the hole, or a balloon may be placed in the maxillary sinus, which lies directly under the orbit. When the balloon is inflated, the contents of the orbit, which have fallen into the maxillary sinus, can be pushed back up into their proper position. Some surgeons use a combination of both of these approaches.

Prevention of eye injuries is much more simple than their repair. The use of safety glasses in industry and in private homes is extremely important. Whenever a person is exposed to a situation that might injure the eye, he should put on safety glasses. Wearing of plastic or shatter-proof glasses is an additional precaution.

The incidence of ocular injury is high, especially in children. It is important to teach children, as well as adults, the hazards of ocular injury and train them to safeguard their eyes. If an eye is injured, immediate and intensive treatment is important. This often restores useful vision.

QUESTIONS

1. What is the most common eye injury?
2. How does patching help a corneal abrasion to heal?
3. What is actinic keratitis?
4. What is the most important thing to do for a chemical burn of the eye?

5. Why is a lye burn of the eye so serious?
6. How may a magnet be helpful to an ophthalmologist?
7. What are some secondary problems that can be caused by a penetrating ocular foreign body?
8. What is a laceration of the globe?
9. How should the layman handle somebody with a suspected lacerated globe?
10. How can a blunt blow to the front of the eye cause damage to the retina?
11. What is a hyphema?
12. How can many serious eye injuries be prevented?

Chapter 13

ANSWERS TO QUESTIONS THAT
ARE FREQUENTLY ASKED

QUESTION: If I wear glasses will I become dependent on them?

ANSWER: One becomes dependent on glasses only if the glasses are beneficial, very much as one becomes dependent on eating, sleeping, and so on. Glasses neither help nor hurt the eyes, they simply enable the person who is wearing them to see more clearly. However, he is not hooked on glasses like a drug user becomes hooked on drugs.

QUESTION: Is a cataract a scum or film over the eye?

ANSWER: A cataract is not a scum or film over the eye; it is simply the clear lens inside of the eye that has become cloudy.

QUESTION: Will eye exercises make my eyes stronger?

ANSWER: Sometimes eye exercises, as supervised by a trained orthoptic technician, are helpful in treating strabismus and perhaps suppression of vision, or early amblyopia in children whose vision has not completely developed. However, most eye exercises designed to make one see better without glasses or to keep the eye muscles strong are neither harmful nor helpful; they are just a waste of time.

QUESTION: My child does not read very well. Is there something wrong with his eyes?

ANSWER: Most reading difficulties in children are not due to poor vision but to a combination of mental, emotional, and other related factors. Many children who have a reading problem have completely normal eyes. Occasionally a child with congenital nystagmus, congenital cataract, or some such maladjustment may have more difficulty seeing the print on the blackboard, but large print material or regular print textbooks held at close range alleviates this condition.

QUESTION: I have frequent headaches. Are my eyes responsible?

ANSWER: Most headaches are not caused by ocular problems. Eye-strain, undetected astigmatism, or squinting may cause slight headache, but this is generally relieved by simply correcting the visual activity that caused it. Of course, eye diseases like iritis or glaucoma may cause considerable pain in the eye and an associated headache. Some migraine headaches may be preceded by visual phenomena such as sparkling lights or small dots bouncing around in front of the field of vision, but this unique event takes place in the occipital lobe of the brain and not in the eye itself. Headaches due to refractive errors can be alleviated by the fitting of proper glasses. Those due to eye pathology will respond to treating the underlying eye disease. But in most instances, headaches are not directly traceable to ophthalmic problems.

QUESTION: Doctor, I see spots in front of my eyes. Is something wrong?

ANSWER: Floaters or spots before the eyes are very frequent, especially in nearsighted people. These are caused by bits of material floating around in the clear vitreous jelly. Occasionally a sudden shower of floaters may signify a broken blood vessel or an impending retinal detachment. Generally a retinal detachment is also accompanied by flashes of light along with the floaters. Anyone with a sudden increase in the number of floaters or experiencing severe flashing lights should have an eye checkup quickly by an ophthalmic surgeon.

QUESTION: Isn't glaucoma a cancer of the eye?

ANSWER: No. Glaucoma has nothing to do with cancer. It is simply an elevated pressure in the eye.

QUESTION: I read about eye transplants. One of my eyes is blind. Could you transplant a new eye to take its place?

ANSWER: There is no such thing as an *eye* transplant. *Corneal* transplant is the only type of transplantation that is performed in ophthalmology. Obviously if the eye is to be removed, the optic nerve has to be cut and all communication with the brain is severed. Now if a new *eye* is transplanted into the empty socket it will have to be reconnected with the brain or it won't function. This means individually reconnecting each nerve fiber cell, which, because it has been cut, has been killed. This type of surgery is impossible at our present level of medical expertise.

QUESTION: Doctor, I see streamers and lines coming out of lights when I drive at night. What causes this?

ANSWER: Lights blurring or bothering you when driving at night is a frequent complication of advancing years. Generally the problem is caused by the lens of the eye becoming more compact and having more and more layers as the years increase. This causes a certain shattering of high contrast lights when the pupil is widely dilated during night driving. It is of little significance except that frequently after this phenomena begins early cataract changes are noted in the lens. There is nothing to do about this condition except to curtail night driving somewhat and have an eye examination.

QUESTION: Doctor, my child reads in very bad light. Doesn't this hurt his eyes?

ANSWER: No. While it is more comfortable to read in a well-lit, glare-free situation, no actual physical damage is done to the eyes by reading under dimly lit conditions.

QUESTION: Doctor, do I have to wear my glasses all the time?

ANSWER: No. Except for some children who need glasses to keep their eyes straight or to keep the vision in the two eyes approximately the same, most people wear glasses to simply improve the clarity of their vision.

QUESTION: Does watching TV hurt my eyes?

ANSWER: No.

QUESTION: Can I use my eyes too much?

ANSWER: No.

QUESTION: I have glaucoma. Can I drink coffee?

ANSWER: Anybody who has glaucoma can have the intraocular pressure of their eyes raised by ingesting large quantities of fluid over a short period of time. However, if their glaucoma has been diagnosed and is in adequate control, drinking coffee or any other fluid in reasonable amounts is perfectly O.K.

QUESTION: If I eat a lot of carrots will it help my eyes? Or, if I take vitamin A, will that help?

ANSWER: The ordinary diet contains a goodly supply of vitamin A. However, in areas of extreme deprivation or in prison camps where inmates are confined for long periods of time, there is a possibility of vitamin A deficiency. However, it is not necessary to consume large amounts of vitamin A. This probably won't hurt anything, but it certainly won't make the eyes any better than under ordinary dietary situations.

QUESTION: I have cataracts. Do I need an operation immediately?

ANSWER: Many people with cataracts never require cataract surgery because their vision remains adequate for their needs during their lifetime. The only time people with cataracts require immediate surgery is when the cataract has reached a state of maturity, threatens to become hypermature or breaks down, causing problems inside the eye. Occasionally a person will develop glaucoma due to a cataract and the treatment for the glaucoma is simply removing the cataract. Most cataracts come on slowly and gradually and can be watched from time to time by a competent ophthalmic surgeon. Generally cataract surgery can be scheduled months in advance.

QUESTION: Will it hurt my eyes if I look directly at the sun or watch an eclipse?

ANSWER: If you look directly at the sun or watch an eclipse of the sun, there is a very good chance that the rays of light focusing on the macular area of the eyes will cause damage to the retinal cells and will result in a permanently scarred macula and a permanent loss of vision. Looking directly at the sun is a very foolish thing to do.

QUESTION: I have been reading about the laser beam in eye surgery. Is it helpful in cataract surgery?

ANSWER: While the laser beam is helpful in retinal detachment surgery and in some diseases of the retina, it is not used to remove the cataract. However, if a clouding of the membrane behind the IOL occurs laser is used to make an opening in the membrane.

QUESTION: Will smoking hurt my eyes?

ANSWER: Tobacco smoke is an irritant to the conjunctiva and will cause a low grade conjunctivitis. Also, people who smoke large quantities of tobacco (cigars and pipes) and consume large quantities of alcohol may get so-called *alcohol-tobacco amblyopia* due to the direct toxic effect of these substances on the cells of the retina.

QUESTION: If I wear the wrong glasses, will it hurt my eyes?

ANSWER: Glasses should be properly prescribed and fitted. If you're wearing the wrong glasses you may experience several difficulties: you may not see as well as you should, you may get some feeling of eyestrain as you try to focus more accurately through the improper glasses. However, wearing the wrong glasses will not damage the eyes.

QUESTION: Will it hurt my eyes to wear sunglasses or tinted glasses?

ANSWER: Some people find wearing sunglasses on bright days more comfortable than going without. However, wearing sunglasses indoors or on dimly lit days is ridiculous. Most people who wear tinted lenses constantly are wearing them more for cosmetic reasons than for eye comfort. However, sunglasses per se, are not harmful.

QUESTION: I work with machinery. Should I wear shatterproof glasses?

ANSWER: Definitely. In fact, all glasses should be made of impact-resistant materials since one of the worst injuries to an eye is being cut by a piece of broken glass. This often results in permanent loss of vision or even loss of the eye and is a very common situation in this country today. The first state law for eye protection in schools became effective in Ohio in August, 1963, and required industry-proved eye protection for all students and teachers using laboratory and shop facilities. Most states now have such a law in effect. I encourage this for everybody, everywhere, regardless of their occupation.

QUESTION: What is micro-surgery?

ANSWER: Micro-surgery is simply surgery performed under an operating microscope. The surgeon and his assistant sit looking through an operating microscope, which is a microscope with a zoom focus lens, a powerful light source, and usually a video camera or a movie camera attached to it. This produces excellent magnification and lighting and many ophthalmic surgeons feel this instrument is invaluable in helping them perform delicate surgical procedures.

QUESTION: I'm about to have a cataract operation, should I have a lens implant?

ANSWER: Yes.

QUESTION: I have trouble reading with my glasses and I find that I can read the small print much easier with a magnifying glass. Is this a good habit?

ANSWER: Many people who are older and experiencing some macular degeneration and perhaps early cataract changes find that the best magnification can be obtained by the use of a magnifying glass. They should be encouraged to use the magnifying glass; it won't hurt their eyes.

QUESTION: Can you recommend a good eye wash?

ANSWER: Cold water from the faucet splashed into and around the eyes two or three times daily, with clean hands, is probably as good an eye wash for general purposes as anything. It can be made a little stronger by using one teaspoonful of table salt to one pint of boiled water. Cool, then bathe the eye from an eye cup.

QUESTION: How often should I have my eyes checked?

ANSWER: Probably every adult over the age of forty should have his eyes checked at least every other year partly for general reasons but more specifically because of the possibility of having glaucoma that is going unnoticed. Children can have their eyes checked less frequently, perhaps every three or four years if there doesn't seem to be any problem. Young adults can also probably go four to five years between eye checks if they are not having any visual problems.

QUESTION: Does crying hurt my eyes?

ANSWER: No. Crying does not in any way hurt your eyes. On the contrary, people who have difficulty crying and suffer from dry eyes are chronically uncomfortable and prone to eye infections and allergies.

QUESTION: Can you tell if someone is dead by looking at his eyes?

ANSWER: If a person is dead, he will have lost all pupillary reflexes and all pain reflexes around the eyes. In addition, doctors with an ophthalmoscope can examine the blood vessels in the back of the eyes. If the blood is beginning to sludge in the blood vessels it is almost a sure sign of death.

QUESTION: Why do my eyes hurt when I come out of the movie theater into the bright daylight?

ANSWER: The pupil dilates and is quite relaxed when you sit in a dark room. Changing suddenly from the dark to the light causes an extreme pupillary constriction which is almost painful for a few moments. Also there is a dazzle phenomena to the retina, which is somewhat uncomfortable.

QUESTION: What should be done in cases of emergency?

ANSWER: 1. *Chemical injuries:* Irrigate the eyes immediately with large amounts of tap water. The most dangerous chemical is lye. Irrigate any lye burn for at least fifteen or twenty minutes with your head held directly under the faucet. Then go to the closest emergency room and seek immediate medical care.

2. *Foreign bodies:* If you suspect that there is a foreign body in your eye, there probably is, and you should see your eye doctor. If you have been involved in a more severe accident, and there is any question that a foreign body may have penetrated inside the eye itself, seek medical attention·immediately. Do not attempt to remove the foreign body. If there is a clean handkerchief or a clean medical dressing available, this can be taped lightly over the eye to afford some protection on your way to the hospital.

3. *Sun-lamp burns:* Sun-lamp burns do not become painful until six to eight hours after exposure to the sun lamp. Then both eyes become extremely irritated and painful. You should have immediate medical attention both for the relief of pain and for protection of possible further damage to the eyes.

4. *Sudden visual loss:* Occasionally people will have sudden transient

loss of vision in one or both eyes or both fields of vision, lasting for a few seconds and not recurring. This is probably of little significance. However, anyone experiencing a sudden loss of vision for more than a few minutes should seek immediate medical attention. This may be due to a blood vessel closing off, or breaking, or it may be due to retinal detachment. It is not at all wise to dally about seeing a physician if your vision in one or both eyes suddenly blacks out.

5. A good *general rule* for any eye emergency is if you don't know what you're doing, don't do it. Simply leave the eye alone and seek immediate attention.

A GLOSSARY OF COMMONLY-USED EYE TERMS

abduction *(ab-duk´shun)*
  Turning outward from axis of body

accommodation *(ah-kom´o-da´shun)*
  Adjustment of the eye for seeing objects at various distances; accomplished by altering the shape of the crystalline lens by action of the ciliary muscle, thus changing its power and focusing a clear image on the retina.

after-image *(af´ter-im´ij)*
  Visual impression which remains after a stimulus is removed

amblyopia ex anopsia *(am-ble-c´pe-ah ex-anop´sia)*
  Amblyopia acquired through lack of use of the eye

aqueous *(ak´we-us)*
  Clear fluid which fills the front part of the eye

asthenopia *(as´the-nc´pi-a)*
  Eye strain caused by fatigue of the internal or external muscles

astigmatism *(ah-stig´mah-tizm)*
  Defective curvature of the refractive surfaces of the eye as a result of which light rays are not sharply focused on the retina for either near or distance

binocular vision *(bin-ok´u-lar)*
  The ability to use the two eyes simultaneously to focus on the same object and to fuse the two images into a single image, which gives a correct interpretation of its solidity and its position in space

blepharitis *(blef-ah-ri´tis)*
  Chronic inflammation of the margins of the eyelids including the hair follicles.

cataract *(kat´ah-rakt)*
  A condition in which the crystalline lens of the eye becomes opaque with consequent loss of visual acuity.

chalazion *(kah-la´ze-on)*

97

Chronic enlargement of one of the meibomian oil glands in the eyelids forming a hard round lump due to blocking of the gland opening

chiasma *(ki-az'ma)*

The crossing of the nerve fibers of the optic nerve

choroiditis *(ko-roid-i'tis)*

Inflammation of the choroid (the blood vessel layer of the eye) due to an infection or allergy

cones and rods

The two types of light-sensitive receptors that are present in the retina and make it possible for it to transmit visual impulses to the brain. Cones are sensitive to the fine detail and color; rods are concerned with motion and vision at low degrees of illumination (as in night vision)

congenital *(kon-jen'i-tal)*

Present at birth

conjunctivitis *(kon-junk'ti-vi'tis)*

An inflammation of the conjunctiva

contact or corneal lenses *(kon'takt, kor'ne-al)*

Lenses so constructed that they fit directly on the eyeball; used for the correction of vision.

convergence *(con-ver'jens)*

The process of directing the visual axes of the two eyes to a near point, with a result that the pupils of the two eyes are closer together, or turned inward.

convergence: near point

The nearest point at which the two eyes can direct their gaze simultaneously; normally about three inches from the nose

corneal graft *(kor'ne-al)*

Operation to restore vision by replacing a section of opaque cornea with transparent corneal tissue from a cadaver.

cycloplegics *(si-klo-ple'jiks)*

A group of drugs, instilled into the eye, which cause temporary paralysis and relaxation of the ciliary muscles, which control accommodation and dilation of the pupil; often used to ascertain the error of refraction

dacryocystitis *(dak're-o-sis-ti'tis)*

Inflammation of the lacrimal sac (tear sac)

diopter *di-op'ter)*

Unit of measurement of strength or refractive power of lenses

diplopia *(di-plo'pe'ah)*
Double vision, i.e. perception of two images of a single object

divergence *(di-ver'jens)*
Simultaneous turning outward of both eyes away from each other

dyslexia *(dis-lek'se-ah)*
Inability to read or understand printed symbols

emmetropia *(em-e-tro'pe-ah)*
Refractive condition of the normal eye, at rest, which brings the image of distant objects to a focus on the retina

enucleation *(e-nu-kle-a'shun)*
Complete surgical removal of the eyeball

esophoria *(es-o-fo're-ah)*
Latent tendency of the eye to turn inward (*see* heterophoria)

esotropia *(es-o-tro'pe-ah)*
An observable turning in of one eye (convergent strabismus or crossed eye)

exophoria *(ek-so-fo're-ah)*
A latent tendency of the eye to turn outward (*see* heterophoria)

exophthalmus *(ek-sof-thal'mos)*
Abnormal protrusion or bulging of the eyeballs from their sockets

extortion *(eks-tor'shun)*
Outward rotation

exotropia *(ek-so-tro'pe-ah)*
(divergent strabismus) Observable turning outward of one eye from the visual axis of the other

Eye Bank
The clearing house for donated eyes

field of vision
The entire area which can be seen at one time by the fixed eye, i.e. without shifting the head or eyes

fluctuating lens myopia *(mi-o'pi-a)*
Swelling of lens fibers because of diabetes

focus *(fo'cus)*
Point to which rays are converted after passing through a lens; focal distance is the distance rays travel after refraction to the point of focus

fovea centralis *(fo've-a sen-tral'is)*
The rodless central area of the retina; fixation point of acute vision

fusion *(fu'-zhun)*
Coordination of the separate images seen by each eye into one

glare

A quality of light which causes discomfort in the eye; it may result from a direct light source within the field of vision or from a reflection of a light source not in the field of vision

glaucoma *(glaw-ko'mah)*

Disease of the eye marked by a mechanical increase in the intraocular pressure causing organic changes in the optic nerve and defects in the visual field.

herpes simplex kerratitis *(her'peez)*

Cold sore on cornea

heterophoria *(het'er-o-fo're-ah)*

A tendency of the eyes to deviate from the normal position for binocular fixation, counterbalanced by simultaneous fixation and fusion (prompted by the desire for single binocular vision). Deviation is not usually apparent, in which case it is called latent heterophoria

heterotropia *(het'er-o-tro'pe-ah)*

Squint, strabismus, cross-eye; when one or more muscles are out of balance, one eye may turn while the other fixes

hordeolum *(hor-de'o-lum)*

A sty; inflammation of one or more of the sweat glands found around the roots of the eyelashes

hydrophthalmus *(hi-drof-thal'mos)*

(congenital glaucoma) A rare congenital defect in which the eyeball is abnormally large as the result of pressure elevation. It is present at birth or develops early in infancy

hyperopia *(hi-per-o'pe-ah)*

Hypermetropia, farsightedness; condition of eye in which light rays from distant objects are brought to focus behind the retina when the eye is at rest

inferior oblique or **trochlear muscle** *(trok'le-er)*

Muscle which tilts the eyeball up and inward

inferior rectus muscle *(rek'tus)*

Muscle of the eye which pulls the eyeball downward

interstitial keratitis *(in-ter-stish'al ker-a-ti'tis)*

A cellular infiltration of the deep layers of the cornea as a result of tuberculosis or syphilis

iridectomy *(ir-i-dek'tom-e)*

Surgery in which a piece of the iris is removed

iris *(i'ris)*

Colored, circular membrane suspended behind the cornea immediately in front of the lens, which regulates the amount of light entering the eye chamber by changing the size of the pupil

iritis *(i-ri'tis)*

Inflammation of the iris; condition marked by pain; inflammation, discomfort from light

keratitis *(ker-a-ti'tis)*

Inflammation of the cornea

lacrimal gland *(lak'ri-mal)*

A gland, located above the outer corner of each eye, which secretes tears

lacrimation *(lak-ri-ma'shun)*

Production of tears

lagophthalmos *(lag-of-thal'mos)*

Inadequate closure of the eyelids

lateral rectus muscle *(rek'tus)*

Muscle of the eye which pulls the eyeball outwards

lens, concave

Lens having power to diverge rays of light; also known as diverging, reducing, negative, or minus lens; denoted by the minus sign

lens, convex

Lens having power to converge rays of light and bring them to a focus; also known as converging, magnifying, hyperopic, or plus lens; denoted by the plus sign

lens, crystalline

A refractive medium having one or both surfaces curved

Lens, IOL *(intra ocular lens)*

A lens which is placed in the eye after a cataract is removed

lumen *(lu'men)*

A unit of measurement of the light output or brightness of light source. Light bulbs are now rated in lumens, in addition to wattage designation

medial rectus muscle *(rek'tus)*

Muscle of the eye which pulls the eyeball inward

microphthalmia *(mi-krof-thal'me-ah)*

Abnormal smallness of the eyes

migraine *(mi'gran)*

A vascular headache complex

myopia *(mi-o'pe-ah)*

A refractive error in which rays of light come to a focus in front of the retina as a result of eyeball being too long from front to back, or having excessive curvature of cornea or lens

myopic *(mi-o'pik)*

Nearsightedness; a condition of the eye in which the point of focus for rays of light from distant objects is in front of the retina

nystagmus *(nis-tag'mus)*

An involuntary movement of the eyeballs rapidly from side to side, up and down, in a rotary motion, or mixed

occlusion *(o-kloo'zhun)*

Act of obscuring the vision of one eye, so as to force the use of the other eye

oculist *(ok'u-list)*

Older term for ophthalmologist

ophthalmia neonatorum *(of-thal'mi-a ne-o-na-to'rum)*

An acute inflammation in the newborn

ophthalmologist *(of-thal-mol'o-jist)*

A physician, an M.D., who specializes in diagnosis and treatment of diseases of the eye.

optic atrophy *(at'ro-fe)*

Wasting away of the optic nerve fibers characterized by pallor of the optic nerve head and accompanied by visual loss

optician *(op-tish'an)*

Technician who grinds lenses, fits them into frames, and adjusts frames to the wearer

optometrist *(op-tom'e-trist)*

A licensed doctor of optometry (O.D.)

orthoptist *(or'thop'tist)*

A person who uses a series of scientifically planned exercises for developing or attempting to restore the normal teamwork of the eyes

peripheral vision *(pe-rif'er-al)*

Ability to perceive presence, motion, or color of objects outside the direct line of vision

phoria *(fo're-ah)*

A latent tendency toward crossed eyes; condition not usually observed; see esophoria, exophoria, and heterophoria

pinguecula *(ping-gwek'u-lah)*

A small, yellowish, often triangular, spot or swelling in the conjunctiva to either side of the cornea, usually on the nasal side; it is not painful; most commonly seen in older people

presbyopia *(pres'be-o'pe-ah)*
Decreased elasticity in the lens of the eye causing some loss of accommodation, and usually seen in older persons

prism *(prizm)*
A wedge-shaped piece of glass or plastic which possesses the power of refracting (bending) rays of light toward its base

pterygium *(te-rij'e-um)*
A condition in which a triangular membrane forms extending from the conjunctiva onto the surface of the cornea

ptosis *(to'sis)*
A drooping of the upper lid due to weakness or paralysis of a portion (or branch) of the third nerve which controls the levator muscle that raises the lid

refraction *(re-frak'shun)*
The bending or deviation of rays of light in passing obliquely from one medium to another of different density; the determination of the refractive errors of the eye and their correction by lenses

refractive error
A defect in the eye's ability to bring light rays to focus on the retina

retinal detachment *(ret'i-nal)*
Separation of the retina from the underlying vascular or choroid layer of the eye breaking connections between the rods and cones and the pigment layer; most often the result of a hole or a tear in the retina

retinitis *(ret-i-ni'tis)*
Inflammation of the retina

retinitis pigmentosa *(pigmento'sa)*
A form of hereditary degeneration of the retina which begins as night blindness, but which produces a gradual loss of vision which may become complete

retrolental fibroplasia *(ret'ro-len'tal fi'bro-pla'zha)*
An opaque membrane seen behind the lens often found in babies born prematurely who have had an excess of oxygen

rod and cones
See cones and rods

rosacea *(ro-za'sha)*
Skin disease which may affect conjunctiva and cornea

sclera *(skle'ra)*

Structure which, with cornea, forms the external coat of the eyeball

scotoma *(sko-to´mah)*

An abnormal blind spot in the field of vision surrounded by an area of normal vision

scotopic vision *(sko-top´ik)*

Seeing with the rods of the eye in dim light; night vision

second sight

Increase in myopia due to early stages of cataract

sphincter muscle *(sfing´ter)*

Muscle which contracts to make the pupil smaller

stereopsis *(ste-re-op´sis)*

Depth perception

strabismus *(strah-biz´mus)*

Manifest deviation of the eyes so that they are not simultaneously directed to the same object; see heterotrophia

stye *(sti)*

Acute inflammation of a sebaccous gland in the eyelid due to infection

superior rectus muscle *(rek´tus)*

Muscle of the eye which pulls the eyeball upwards

sympathetic ophthalmitis *(of´-thal-mi´tis)*

Severe inflammation of one eye due to infection in the other eye

telescopic lenses

Special lenses for persons with advanced degrees of sight impairment; two lenses, properly ground, and mounted with a short distance between them to form a sort of telescope

tonometer *(to-nom´e-ter)*

Instrument used in measuring tension or pressure in order to check for glaucoma

trachoma *(trah-ko´mah)*

Chronic contagious conjunctivitis producing loss of vision

trichromatic *(tri-kro-mat´ik)*

Having or pertaining to normal color vision

trifocals *(tri-fo´kalz)*

A bifocal lens with an added lens to allow vision at intermediate distances

unilateral aphakia *(a-fa´kiah)*

Case where the cataract has been removed from one eye, the other eye having good vision

vernal catarrh *(ver´nal ka-tar´)*

An unpleasant type of allergic conjunctivitis
vision *(vizh'un)*
The ability to see and interpret what is seen
visual acuity *(ah-ku'i-te)*
Sharpness of vision, the ability of the eye to distinguish detail

INDEX

107